THE BIOCHEMIC HANDBOOK

An introduction to the cellular therapy and practical application
of the twelve tissue cell-salts in accordance with the biochemic
system of medicine of Dr W. H. Schuessler.

THE
BIOCHEMIC
HANDBOOK

Revised by Colin B. Lessell

M.B., B.S.(Lond.), B.D.S.(Lond.), M.R.C.S.(Eng.), L.R.C.P.(Lond.)

THORSONS PUBLISHERS LIMITED
Wellingborough, Northamptonshire

This edition, completely revised and reset, 1984

© THORSONS PUBLISHERS LIMITED 1984

British Library Cataloguing in Publication Data

Lessell, Colin B.
  The biochemic handbook.—Completely rev.
and reset ed.
  1. Medicine, Biochemic
  I. Title   II. Goodwin, J. S. Biochemic
  handbook
  615.5'8   RZ412

  ISBN 0-7225-0891-3

Printed and bound in Great Britain

Contents

An Introduction to Biochemics

The Biochemic system of medicinal therapy is to be attributed to Dr Wilhelm H. Scheussler of Oldenburg, Germany. His major work in this respect was carried out between the years 1872 and 1898. Following his death, early in 1898, further development of his system was not arrested, but continued through the efforts of a multitude of homoeopathic physicians. Its demonstrable efficacy in the treatment of disease has enabled it to survive into the modern era, and it stands as a fitting monument to its illustrious founder.

Dr Scheussler believed that disease process was always associated with deficiency of one or more inorganic substances, which he termed *tissue-salts*. The twelve *tissue-salts* of Scheussler are:

1. Calcium fluoride (*Calc. Fluor.*)
2. Calcium phosphate (*Calc. Phos.*)
3. Calcium sulphate (*Calc. Sulph.*)
4. Ferric (Iron) phosphate (*Ferr. Phos.*)
5. Potassium chloride (*Kali. Mur.*)
6. Potassium phosphate (*Kali. Phos.*)
7. Potassium sulphate (*Kali. Sulph.*)
8. Magnesium phosphate (*Mag. Phos.*)
9. Sodium chloride (*Nat. Mur.*)
10. Sodium phosphate (*Nat. Phos.*)
11. Sodium sulphate (*Nat. Sulph.*)
12. Silicon dioxide (*Silica*)

In Scheusslerian theory, each deficiency is characterized by certain objective and subjective symptoms, and is thus readily identified. The deficient tissue-salt, or salts, must then be *replaced* by the administration in *minute* dosage of special preparations thereof.

With increased scientific knowledge, however, we are now aware that Scheusslerian theory is incorrect in certain respects. Whilst these biochemic remedies may, even today, be selected according to the symptoms of the individual patient, and achieve appropriate therapeutic results, just as described by Scheussler himself, the dosages themselves are too small to replace any deficiency *directly*. Whilst not refuting the clinical efficacy of his methods, are we to assume, therefore, that Scheussler was entirely misguided in his scientific basis?

Fortunately he may be largely vindicated in this respect by considering the discoveries of modern biochemistry, the study of chemical processes within the living body. For example, the remedy *Mag. Phos.* is a key remedy in the treatment of menstrual cramps in women. It is now known that this condition may be associated with magnesium deficiency. Having stated that the dosages utilized in the biochemic system are too small to act as magnesium replacement therapy, how then could *Mag. Phos.* act? One distinct possibility is that this biochemic preparation is capable of influencing the way in which magnesium is distributed throughout the body, and thus serves to rectify any magnesium imbalances, and the symptomatic consequences of the latter.

It would also seem that the biochemic remedies are able to treat *excesses* of substances within the body. *Nat. Mur.*, prepared from salt, may, in certain circumstances, be of use in preventing excessive sodium retention and thus, secondarily, may control fluid retention. *Calc. Fluor.* is often of service in the reduction of bony overgrowth, as in some types of osteoarthritis, where, effectively, there is a local surplus of calcium salts.

Viewed overall, the biochemic tissue-salts may be regarded as a group of *regulatory* remedies, rather than a group concerned merely with the rectification of deficiency states. That is to say, they influence the distribution of ions (electrically charged atoms and molecules) and molecules throughout the body.

Hopefully, having accepted the concept of deficiency or excess in disease, the enquiring reader might now well suggest that dietetic modification must surely be the simplest remedy for such disturbances. Indeed, one frequently meets cases in clinical practice where this is so. A child with a very low calcium intake will develop bony deformities, and calcium must be increased in the diet. An adult with high blood pressure consequent upon the consumption of vast amounts of salt must have his salt intake reduced. To neglect the matter of diet in these cases would be foolhardy.

However, in many instances the problem is one of improper distribution or utilization of substances in the body, thus creating *localized* deficiencies or excesses, and even the most radical dietetic changes will not improve the patient's lot. Here, the biochemic tissue-salts may be of great service.

In other instances, improvement is secured by a combination of dietetic modification (which may include the provision of vitamin or mineral supplements), *and* the application of biochemic remedies, to the greater advantage of the patient. It is always wise to remember that the use of the biochemics alone is inadvisable in the face of gross nutritional excesses or deficiencies. As explained, they are *not* a replacement therapy. In anaemia of pregnancy, it is initially prudent to ensure that there is an adequate intake of iron, Vitamin C (which facilitates iron absorption from the gut), and folic acid. This we may do by administering brewer's yeast, and advising an increased intake of foods containing Vitamin C, such as fresh fruit. Having achieved this, and still the patient is anaemic, then we may justifiably administer *Ferr. Phos.*

Whilst Scheussler fervently maintained that the biochemic system was quite different in principle from the Hahnemannian system of homoeopathy, it is now generally accepted by homoeopathic physicians that it is, in reality, an extension of the homoeopathic system, a fact which does nothing towards diminishing its value. The regulatory function of the biochemic remedies is utterly consistent with the mode of action of many established homoeopathic remedies. In the second place, there is Scheussler's assertion that, whereas classical homoeopathic remedies are selected on the basis of the *Law of Similars*, the biochemic remedies are primarily selected on the known chemical structure of the tissues. This point requires some expansion.

Essentially the *Law of Similars* states that the ability of a drug to induce disease in the healthy determines its ability (in reduced dosage) to cure similar disease in the sick. Thus, the drug *Belladonna* (Deadly Nightshade) induces in the healthy: dry mouth, flushed face, and delirium. Hence its use in the treatment of infective disease of childhood, characterized by dry mouth, flushed face, and delirium.

By contrast, the biochemic tissue salt *Kali. Phos.* is used in the treatment of diseases of the nervous system because this inorganic salt is found in large quantities in the ash that remains after combustion of nerve tissue, a supposed deficiency of this salt being associated with such diseases.

However, Dr H. C. Allen has demonstrated that the use of *Kali. Phos.* in diseases of the nervous system is consistent with the *Law of Similars*, since it is capable of producing similar symptoms in healthy subjects. That is to say, *Kali. Phos.* is *homoeopathic* to certain types of nervous disease. That Scheussler's rationale for the use of this remedy was different, does not alter this fact. Similarly, that the biochemics are homoeopathic remedies does not necessarily negate the fundamentals of biochemic theory. The two views are compatible.

Furthermore, the mode of preparation of the tissue salts for administration to patients is essentially the same as that for classical insoluble homoeopathic remedies, *viz.* serial dilution and trituration. One part of the salt is mixed with nine parts of lactose (milk-sugar), and the resultant mixture subjected to a vigorous grinding process, termed *trituration*. This is the *first decimal* potency, labelled 1x. One part of the 1x potency is mixed with nine parts of lactose, and triturated. This is the *second decimal* potency, labelled 2x. One part of the 2x potency is similarly diluted and triturated with lactose to yield the *third decimal* potency, labelled 3x. The notation 'x' is taken from the Latin numeral X (= 10), referring to serial dilutions of 1/10. The dilution and trituration process may be repeated an indefinite number of times in the manner described, but seldom is it necessary to continue beyond a decimal potency of 12x. The most commonly utilized potency is 6x (dilution of one part of tissue-salt per million).

The combined process of serial dilution, with trituration at each stage is termed *potentization*. Trituration, the delivery of mechanical energy to the lactose-tissue salt mixture is vital for the development of medicinal action. It is believed that the mechanical energy so delivered causes the release of electromagnetic energy from the salt, and characteristic of it. This energy is then either held by the molecules of the lactose, or, more likely, by water molecules dispersed throughout the lactose. Generally speaking, an optimal amount of energy is developed by the sixth decimal stage of potentization (6x).

In order to render the *potentized* powder suitable for easy administration, it is compressed into small friable pellets, or small tablets. These readily dissolve either on or under the tongue. Always remember, however, that babies may inhale such pellets, and this is avoided by crushing the pellets on a spoon into a fine powder for direct administration.

Since biochemic tissue-salts *trigger* healing reactions in the body, there is no point in exceeding the usual specified dosages, *viz.* four pellets for an adult, and two for a child. No greater effect can be achieved by administering forty pellets simultaneously, rather than the numbers stated. Furthermore, no harm will be done by such wasteful behaviour, except to one's pocket, since the dilutions involved are considerable. In order to reinforce medicinal action, one must repeat the specified dosages at more frequent intervals; indeed, as often as once every twenty minutes.

As with homoeopathic remedies in general, certain precautions should be taken to ensure efficacy. No food or drink should be consumed within fifteen minutes of taking a remedy. Similarly, cleaning one's teeth should be avoided in this time interval. All tissue salts should be kept in tightly stoppered containers, away from daylight, perfumes and other aromatic substances. Handling the remedies directly should be avoided, except to take the required dose. They should not be transferred to any containers other than those of issue.

The biochemic tissue-salts may be used to treat both acute (short-lived) disease, such as measles, and chronic (prolonged) disease, such as arthritis. With regard to infections, be they viral or bacterial, they work by encouraging the bodily reaction to the infecting organism, rather than upon the infecting organisms themselves. Whilst the reader may assume that they are an extremely safe form of therapy, it is necessary, however, to make some important observations.

Just occasionally, the patient's condition appears to worsen after taking tissue-salts. This is termed a *homoeopathic aggravation* or *healing crisis*. It is due to slight overpromotion of the healing process. Should this occur during the treatment of an acute illness (e.g. mumps), administration of the remedy should immediately be discontinued, in order to allow the body to enter a *healing phase*. In most instances, following this healing crisis, the patient will then go to rapid cure. In some cases, though improvement occurs, it is short of cure, and the services of a homoeopathic physician may be required to complete the process. With these comments born in mind, no anxiety should be felt on the part of the user.

In the treatment of chronic disease (e.g. chronic sinusitis), a healing crisis may also occur. Whilst rarely it may happen in sensitive subjects within a few days of commencing therapy, it may be delayed for several weeks. It is often caused by too frequent repetition of dosage. The remedy should be immediately discontinued, and the patient allowed to enter a healing phase. Should the patient's condition warrant further medication with the same tissue-salt, it may be cautiously restarted with a reduced frequency of dose repetition.

Whilst the applicability of a particular biochemic remedy is determined by the individual symptoms of the patient, it is now possible to purchase special mixtures of various tissue-salts in order to facilitate prescribing for the novice. Newcomers to the biochemic system will find the prescription of these mixtures a relatively simple matter.

From the homoeopathic point of view, the biochemic tissue-salts are a group of remedies, safe for home use, provided the matter of healing crisis is understood, which, as I have said, is relatively rare with the biochemics, in any event. They are not only safe, they are extremely valuable. However, the biochemic system of medicine is not a complete system in itself. It cannot cure all disease. Whilst many patients derive great benefit, others are disappointed with the results. Such failure may be due to unidentified nutritional problems, or poor remedy selection on the part of the patient. Alternatively, it may be due to the fact that homoeopathic remedies of a more deep-acting nature are required. In the case of failure, the patient should seek the services of a homoeopathic physician.

Whereas drugs may reduce the efficacy of the biochemic remedies, the biochemics have no adverse inter-reaction with drugs. Whilst not ideal to take drugs at the same time as tissue-salts, since the curative ability of the latter might be inhibited, all patients must be advised to maintain their prescribed drug therapy until a physician can be consulted.

DR COLIN B. LESSELL

The Twelve Tissue-Salts

1. CALC. FLUOR.
   (*calcium fluoride*)
2. CALC. PHOS.
   (*Calcium phosphate*)
3. CALC. SULPH.
   (*Calcium sulphate*)
4. FERR. PHOS.
   (*Phosphate of Iron*)
5. KALI. MUR.
   (*Potassium chloride*)
6. KALI. PHOS.
   (*Potassium phosphate*)
7. KALI. SULPH.
   (*Potassium sulphate*)
8. MAG. PHOS.
   (*Magnesium phosphate*)
9. NAT. MUR.
   (*Sodium chloride*)
10. NAT. PHOS.
    (*Sodium phosphate*)
11. NAT. SULPH.
    (*Sodium sulphate*)
12. SILICA
    (*Silicon dioxide*)

Their Place and Function in the Human Economy

CALC. FLUOR. (Calcium fluoride)

This tissue-salt is indicated wherever symptoms are due to a relaxed condition e.g. enlarged and varicose veins, with associated ulcerations and eczema, piles, sluggish circulation. It should also be considered for constipation when due to relaxed muscles of the rectum. A backache with dragging down bearing pain calls for this remedy, and so does chronic synovitis. A useful alternative remedy to Kali. Sulph. and Silica in the treatment of brittle nails.

   Calc. Fluor. is also of value for diseases affecting the surface of the bones, cracks and cuts in the skin. A poor condition of the enamel of the teeth calls for this tissue-salt.

Note: *Calcium fluoride should not be confused with Sodium fluoride which is used for fluoridating water supplies. This has known risks.*

CALC. PHOS. (Calcium phosphate)

Calc. Phos. promotes healthy cellular activity and restores tone to weakened organs and tissues. It assists digestion and assimilation and is a valuable tonic. *Calc. Phos.* is indicated in the treatment of simple anaemia in conjunction with *Ferr. Phos.* In such cases there are often spasms and pains accompanied by sensations of coldness and numbness. If the circulation is slow and retarded then *Calc. Phos.* is called for. It is of value in the treatment of chilblains. Senile itching of the skin (pruritus) points to *Calc. Phos.* in alternation with *Kali. Phos.* It should also be considered for enlarged tonsils, and nasal polypi.

   Calc. Phos. is a useful intercurrent remedy as it assists the action of a more directly indicated tissue-salt and thus produces more rapid results.

CALC. SULPH. (Calcium sulphate)

Calc. Sulph. is a 'blood purifier' and healer. *Calc. Sulph.* cleans out the accumulation of non-functional, organic matter in the tissues and causes infiltrated parts to discharge their contents readily, throwing-off decaying organic matter, so that it may not lie dormant or slowly decay and thus injure the surrounding tissues.

   Calc. Sulph. is indicated in conditions arising from impurities in the blood stream. It supplements the action of *Kali. Mur.* in the treatment of catarrh, acne, etc., and it should always be given when 'pimples' occur in adolescence and for gumboils.

   Calc. Sulph. has been found of value in the treatment of frontal headaches and neuralgias in the elderly.

FERR. PHOS. (Iron phosphate)

Ferr. Phos. is the pre-eminent Biochemic First Aid. It gives strength and toughness to the circular walls of the blood vessels, especially the arteries. Freely circulating, oxygen-rich blood is essential to health and life and for this reason *Ferr. Phos.* should always be considered, as a supplementary remedy, no matter what other treatment may be indicated by the symptoms.

Congestion, inflammatory pain, high temperature, quickened pulse, all call for *Ferr. Phos.* This tissue-salt can be given with advantage in the early stage of acute disorders, and it should be administered at frequent intervals until the inflammatory symptoms subside. It is also indicated where there is a lack of red blood corpuscles, as in anaemia. It is an excellent remedy for ailments associated with advancing years and it is one of the most frequently needed remedies in the treatment of children's ailments. *Ferr. Phos.* should also be thought of as a first aid in cases of muscular strains, sprains, etc.

Note: *Ferr. Phos. is in no sense an iron tonic. In its potentised or biochemic form this tissue-salt has none of the disadvantages in ordinary iron medicines. It is easily and quickly assimilated by the blood.*

KALI. MUR. (Potassium chloride)

Soft glandular swellings call for this remedy; also chronic rheumatic swellings. Its action is complementary to that of *Calc. Sulph.*, as both remedies are concerned with cleansing and purifying the blood. It is of particular value in the treatment of infantile eczema. In alternation with *Ferr. Phos.* it is frequently needed for the treatment of children's ailments.

Kali. Mur. is the remedy for thick, white fibrinous discharges. Other prominent symptoms are a white-coated tongue and light-coloured stools (lack of bile). Torpidity of the liver is another indication. In alternation with *Ferr. Phos.* it is indicated in the treatment of inflammatory diseases, particularly those affecting the respiratory system — coughs, colds, sore throats, tonsilitis, bronchitis, etc. *Kali. Mur.* is concerned with digestion. The symptoms may be worse after eating fatty or rich foods and there may be lack of appetite. It is the inorganic analogue of the homoeopathic remedy *Pulsatilla.*

KALI. PHOS. (Potassium phosphate)

Kali. Phos. is indicated for the treatment of nervous headaches, nervous dyspepsia, sleeplessness, depression, languid weariness, lowered vitality, 'grumpiness' and many other conditions. *Kali. Phos.* is not merely a pick-me-up, it has a wide and powerful influence on the bodily functions. It covers those ailments comprehended by the term 'nerves'. *Kali. Phos.* is indicated in the treatment of shingles, to correct the underlying nervous condition. It is helpful for the relief of nervous asthma, in conjunction with *Mag. Phos.*, and insomnia when of nervous origin also calls for these two tissue-salts.

KALI. SULPH. (Potassium sulphate)

This tissue-salt has a special affinity for those cells forming the lining of the skin and those forming the internal mucous lining of all internal organs. *Kali. Sulph.* treats chilliness, flashes of heat, pains in limbs which move from place to place.

Kali Sulph. is the function remedy of the epidermis and of the epithelium: yellow slimy deposit on the tongue, yellowish or greenish discharge from any of the mucous surfaces and epithelial or epidermal scaling. Hence *Kali. Sulph.* is required for certain forms of catarrh and skin troubles with scaling. It is of value in the treatment of psoriasis and athlete's foot. Brittle nails call for *Kali. Sulph.* (*also Silica*). With *Silica* and *Nat. Mur.* it helps to maintain the hair in a healthy state.

MAG. PHOS. (Magnesium phosphate)

Mag. Phos. is known as the anti-spasmodic tissue-salt. Its main function is in connection with the nervous system where it supplements the action of *Kali. Phos. Mag. Phos.* is quick to relieve pain, especially cramping, shooting, darting or spasmodic pains.

Mag. Phos. is indicated for nerve pains, such as neuralgia, neuritis, sciatica and headaches accompanied by shooting, darting stabs of pain. It relieves muscular twitching, cramps, hiccups, convulsive fits of coughing and those sudden, sharp twinges of pain.

Note: *Mag. Phos. will often act more rapidly when the tablets are taken with a sip of hot water.*

NAT. MUR. (Sodium chloride)

Excessive moisture or excessive dryness in any part of the system is a clear indication for *Nat. Mur.* The resulting symptoms are many and varied but always, underlying them, will be found this predominant condition of too much or too little water. Here are some typical symptoms:

Low spirits, with a feeling of hopelessness; headache with constipation; difficult stools, with rawness and soreness of the anus; colds with discharge of watery mucus and sneezing; dry, painful nose and throat symptoms; water-brash due to gastric fermentation with slow digestion, the food remains too long in the stomach; great thirst; toothache and facial neuralgia with flow of tears and saliva; eyes weak, the wind causes them to water; hay fever, drowsiness with muscular weakness; chafing of the skin; unrefreshing sleep, tired in the morning; loss of taste and smell; craving for salt and salty foods; stings and bites of insects — apply locally as soon as possible, see directions (external application).

An important function of *Nat. Mur.* is to regulate the production of hydrochloric acid. Too little acid means slow digestion.

Furthermore, the tissue-salt *Nat. Mur.* can be used with advantage in cases when a salt-free diet is recommended.

Approximately two-thirds of the body is composed of water; hence the vital role played by *Nat. Mur.*, the water distributor, in all the life processes.

NAT. PHOS. (Sodium phosphate)

This tissue-salt is an acid neutraliser. An acid state gives rise to rheumatic troubles, digestive upsets, intestinal disorders, and has an adverse effect upon assimilation.

Nat. Phos. helps to regulate the consistency of the bile and is one of the remedies indicated in the treatment of jaundice, colic, sick headaches, and gastric disturbances.

One of the functions of *Nat. Phos.* is that of promoting the absorption of water, as a result of the decomposition of lactic acid. This function is quite distinct from that of *Nat Mur.* which distributes water, and *Nat. Sulph.* which eliminates surplus water from the body. These three tissue-salts control the behaviour of the body fluids.

Nat. Phos. serves to emulsify fatty acids; it is indicated in the treatment of dyspeptic conditions due to eating fatty or greasy foods. Think of *Nat. Phos.* when uric acid becomes deposited around the joints and tissues giving rise to stiffness, pain and swelling.

All exudations are creamy golden-yellow and the tongue is similarly coated.

NAT. SULPH. (Sodium sulphate)

Nat. Sulph. regulates the density of the intercellular fluids (fluids which bathe the tissue-cells) by eliminating excess water. This tissue-salt largely controls the healthy functioning of the liver; it ensures an adequate supply of free-flowing, healthy bile, so necessary for the later stages of digestion. The removal of poison-charged fluids, which are the normal result of the chemical exchanges constantly taking place in the tissue-cells, is brought about by the action of *Nat. Sulph.* If conditions arise which allow these waste fluids to accumulate in the blood and tissues, auto-intoxication (self-poisoning) is the result.

Nat. Sulph. ensures the disposal of these poison charged fluids and its importance in the treatment of rheumatic ailments is therefore self-evident.

Nat. Sulph. is indicated in the treatment of ailments affecting the liver, e.g. biliousness. Sandy deposits in the urine, watery infiltrations, a brownish-green coating of the tongue and a bitter taste in the mouth are some of the symptoms. It is the principal remedy in the treatment of influenza, eliminating the excess of toxic fluids from the system.

SILICA (Silicon dioxide)

The action of *Silica* is deep and long-lasting, and it is indicated in imperfectly nourished constitutions where there is a history of deficient assimilation.

Silica acts more upon the organic substances of the body, involving particularly the bones, joints, glands and skin and is indicated wherever there is pus formation or threatened suppuration, e.g. abcesses, boils, gumboils, styes, etc. It is useful in the treatment of tonsillitis when pus has begun to form. Brittle nails and an impoverished condition of the hair need this tissue-salt.

In cases of checked perspiration, *Silica* restores the activity of the skin and it is also the remedy for offensive perspiration.

Silica can dissolve the accumulation of urates lodging around the joints and muscles which can occur in rheumatic troubles. *Silica* treats poor memory, slow and difficult thought, and absent mindedness. Elderly people have a general need for *Silica*.

Selecting the Remedy
and Directions

The key to success in using the Schuessler therapy is the accurate linking of the symptoms with the appropriate tissue-salt. Symptoms are significant pointers to the tissue-salts needed in any given case. Each of the tissue-salts has its own distinct symptoms 'picture', i.e., the spasms, cramps and neuralgias of *Mag. Phos.*, acidity which points to *Nat. Phos.*, excess dryness or watery discharges which call for *Nat. Mur.* and so on.

Directions
Definitions: 'Acute' means of sudden onset and short duration. 'Chronic' means of long continuance, lingering. A 'chronic' ailment may have 'acute' phases and for such phases the directions for acute conditions will apply.

Dose
In general, an adult dose is four tablets, children two tablets. The tablets should be dissolved on the tongue, or in the case of very young children, may be given dissolved in a little warm water.

Frequency of Dose
In chronic cases, three doses daily will suffice, but for acute conditions, a dose should be taken every half hour until relief is obtained; thereafter the frequency of dose should be gradually reduced to three times daily.

Alternate Remedies
When more than one remedy is required, it is usual for these to be taken in rotation daily, the frequency of dose depending on the acute or chronic nature of the ailment. On the other hand the predominating

symptoms should be treated first; so try to balance the two to the best advantage.

Intercurrent Remedies

These are remedies, while of secondary importance, which have some bearing on a particular case. Such a remedy would be required where there is some underlying problem such as acidity (*Nat. Phos.*) anaemia (*Calc. Phos.*) nerve weakness (*Kali. Phos.*) and so on. Intercurrent remedies assist the action of the principal remedy or remedies by correcting any secondary condition which may have a retarding effect on the general treatment.

Note: *Although when more than one tissue-salt is required it is usual for these to be taken in rotation, the convenience of a simultaneous dose has obvious advantages, and in many cases results come fully up to expectations.*

Changing the Remedy

In the treatment of some ailments, particularly those of an acute kind, differing symptoms may make their appearance during the course of treatment, and in such cases the remedies should be changed or supplemented in accordance with the variation of the symptoms at each successive stage.

Take the common cold as an example. This usually begins with a feeling of stuffiness, congestion and sometimes feverish state. So in this early stage *Ferr. Phos.* and *Kali. Mur.* are required. This first stage is quite often followed by a watery discharge, a clear pointer to the need of the tissue-salt concerned with excessive moisture *Nat. Mur.*, which should be substituted for *Ferr. Phos.* and *Kali. Mur.* Subsequently, the watery discharge could change to a thick mucous discharge calling for *Calc. Sulph.* or *Kali. Sulph.*, in place of *Nat. Mur.* Finally when the cold has cleared up a short course of *Calc. Phos.* is recommended.

External Application

For dry application a few tablets may be crushed and the powder applied direct to the affected part. This is the usual method of dealing with cuts and abrasions (*Ferr. Phos.*), after the injured part has been cleansed.

As a lotion, dissolve ten tablets in half a tumbler of water, which has previously been boiled and allowed to cool. This lotion should be dabbed on the affected part.

Hymosa Balm is one of New Era Laboratories Ltd., of 39 Wales Farm Road W3 6XH, proprietary Biochemic preparations. It is a mild, antiseptic skin-balm for soothing and healing minor skin ailments. Selected biochemic tissue-salts are incorporated in a smooth non-greasy, colourless base. It is a 'must' for 'nappy rash'.

Elasto Nature Salve is also a New Era product. It supplements the action of the appropriate tissue-salt in the treatment of chilblains, cracks in the skin, varicose eczema and ulcers.

The Application of the Twelve Tissue-Salts

Abscesses and Boils

An acute abscess is one which develops rapidly, beginning as a sore spot in some part of the body, becoming hard, inflamed, painful and filled with pus. When pus formation has occurred it is an indication that the white blood corpuscles have successfully overcome the invading micro-organisms. There may be some fever. Hot fomentations will help to relieve the pain, which subsides when the abscess bursts. Boils resemble abscesses, but usually come in crops. Meticulous cleanliness of the affected area is important in preventing the spread of infection. The action of *Silica* helps the abscess to ripen. A lowered state of health is sometimes a predisposing factor and in such cases a course of *Calc. Phos.* is indicated.

BIOCHEMIC TREATMENT

Ferr. Phos.   First or inflammatory stage, when there is heat, pain, congestion and fever. Given early in alternation with *Kali. Mur.* it will often prevent swelling and suppuration (formation of pus).

Kali. Mur.   For the swelling, before pus has begun to form (alternate with *Ferr. Phos.*).

Silica.   After *Kali. Mur.*, when swelling becomes soft and pus has commenced to form. It will assist suppuration, cause the abscess to ripen and often break without surgical interference. Should also be given after the abscess has broken and is discharging its contents.

Calc. Sulph.   After *Silica*, if the discharge continues too long and the wound refuses to heal owing to a torpidity of the tissues.

Calc. Fluor.   When the suppurative process affects the bone. When the abscess has a hard, callous edge.

Acidity

Acidity is a somewhat loose term indicating that the blood, or one or more of the secretions, is less alkaline than it should be. This excess of acid gives rise to many distressing symptoms. There may be gastric disturbance, irritation of the skin and mucous membranes, impoverishment of the blood, palpitation of the heart, twinges of rheumatism, headache on the top of the head with a sense of fullness, a persistent feeling of tiredness and other symptoms of disturbed metabolism. Whenever signs of acidity make their appearance the principal remedy, *Nat. Phos.*, should be given — irrespective of any other tissue-salt which may be indicated — as this acid state, if allowed to persist, will hamper the action of other tissue-salts.

BIOCHEMIC TREATMENT

Nat. Phos.   The principal remedy whenever symptoms of acidity are present.

Nat. Sulph.   This tissue-salt is one of the alkaline sulphates and it may be used to supplement the action of *Nat. Phos.*

Silica.   Dyspepsia with eructations, heartburn, chilliness. In alternation with *Nat Phos*.

Mag. Phos.   Burning, tasteless eructations, relieved by drinking hot water. Flatulence with distension of the stomach, belching gas and full sensation in the abdomen. *See also Combination C.*

Anaemia

Anaemia is a lowering of the quality of the blood. The blood cells may be too few in number or the oxygen-carrying red constituents of the blood cells may be deficient. Anaemia may result directly from a loss of blood. By giving the needed tissue-salts the blood can usually be restored to its normal amount and quality. Foods rich in vitamins such as red meats, liver, milk, eggs and green vegetables should be included in the diet. Fresh air and sunshine are also recommended.

BIOCHEMIC TREATMENT

Calc. Phos.   The principal remedy to provide new blood-cells. Especially useful to anaemic children and during convalescence.

Ferr. Phos.   Helps in the formation of red blood by bringing oxygen to the new blood-cells.

Nat. Mur. When the blood is thin and watery with depression of spirits and prostration. *Nat. Mur.* is an important remedy in the treatment of anaemia.

Nat. Phos. Useful as an intercurrent remedy and when an acid condition prevails.

Note: *Unlike iron tonics the tissue-salt Ferr. Phos. is immediately assimilated into the system.*

Arthritis

Arthritis is a disease affecting the structure in and about the joints. There is pain, swelling and redness of the affected joints. The condition usually begins in the small joints of the hands, especially the fingers. Subsequently other joints are involved. With recurrent attacks the joints tend to become swollen and fixed. In comparison with the swelling of the joints there is wasting of the surrounding muscle.

Osteoarthritis is another form of arthritis. It is a common disorder of the joints. It is characterized by the gradual destruction of the central part of the cartilage lining the affected joint. There can be changes in bone structure that could include new bone formation which may occur in the form of spurs (an abnormal projection of bone). In advanced cases surgery may be employed.

BIOCHEMIC TREATMENT

Ferr. Phos. In acute attacks with fever, inflammation of the joint which is swollen and red. Painful joints aggravated by motion.

Nat. Phos. When there are acid conditions. In alternation with *Nat. Sulph.*

Nat. Mur. When there is creaking of the joints.

Mag. Phos. Of possible value, in alternation with *Calc. Phos.*, for the relief of pain in osteoarthritis.

See also Zief.

Asthma

Asthma is a disorder of respiration characterized by severe paroxysms of difficult breathing, usually followed by a period of complete relief, with recurrence of the attacks at more or less frequent intervals. The term is often incorrectly employed in reference to states of embarrassed respiration, which are plainly due to permanent organic disease within the chest, and which have none of the distinctive characteristics of true asthma.

Asthma manifests itself by spasmodic contraction of the smaller bronchial tubes. It is this narrowing of the bronchial tubes, often accentuated by swelling of the lining epithelium, that is responsible for the great difficulty in breathing which is the characteristic feature of the condition. There are a large number of substances to which the asthmatic subject may be hypersensitive, contact with which is responsible for an attack. These include pollens; the emanations of certain animals such as cats, dogs, horses, etc.; certain articles of diet; bacteria. The discovery of the substance to which the individual is susceptible may sometimes be difficult.

In many cases the specific susceptibility may be enhanced by some non-specific condition, such as emotional disturbance, indigestion or an infection such as a sore throat or a 'cold in the head'. There is yet another group of asthmatic subjects in whom the asthma is due to some chronic or repeated infection, such as attacks of tonsillitis, sinusitis, or nasal catarrh.

Some alleviation of the symptoms may be obtained with the use of the appropriate tissue-salt.

BIOCHEMIC TREATMENT

Kali. Phos.   Is the chief remedy for the oppressed breathing in frequent doses during attacks. Nervous asthma; asthma from taking the least food; nervous system depressed.

Kali. Mur.   Asthma when derangements of the stomach are present, white coated tongue, costive bowels, sluggish liver. Expectoration is thick, white, tough mucus, hard to cough up. Alternate with *Kali. Phos.* for the breathing.

Mag. Phos.   Asthma with troublesome flatulence or constrictive sensation in the chest. Spasms of the bronchial muscles with paroxysmal dry tickling cough and difficulty in lying down. Alternate with *Kali. Phos.*

Nat. Mur.   Asthma with expectoration of clear, frothy mucus, watery discharges from the eyes and nose. Alternate with *Kali. Phos.*

Calc. Phos.   Intercurrently with the indicated remedies in all cases.

Asthma in children, mucus clear and tough. Bronchial asthma, with *Kali. Sulph.*
Nat. Sulph.   Asthma worse in damp weather or wet surroundings, greenish-yellow coating on the tongue, expectoration greenish and copious.

Backache

Many people have an aching pain in the back. Pain, stiffness or tenderness in the back is a symptom to be met with a number of different diseases. In rheumatism, chronic or acute, there may be much pain and stiffness. Pain in the back about the level of the waist is very often due to spinal disease, or it may be due to kidney trouble. Lumbago is a very common form of backache which is always made worse by stooping.

In women, the pain may be due to a disorder of the reproductive organs. In such cases the pain is usually felt low down in the back. There are, however, many women who suffer from pain in the small of the back without any sign of disease and who are otherwise perfectly well.

BIOCHEMIC TREATMENT
Calc. Fluor.   Dragging pain in the lower part of the back, particularly when associated with displacement of the female organs, or with haemorrhoids.
Ferr. Phos.   Acute lumbago, pain in muscles, especially when in motion.
Mag. Phos.   Neuralgic pains along the spine. Pains are sharp and shooting, relieved by heat but not by rest.
Kali. Phos.   Backache aggravated by motion. Where there is underlying nervous tension.
Calc. Phos.   Pain in the back with coldness and numbness along the spine.
Nat. Sulph.   Rheumatic pain in the back, worse in damp weather and at night.
Nat. Mur.   Pains in the small of the back relieved by lying on something hard. Weak back worse in the morning.
See also Combination G.

Bed Wetting (see **Urinary Disorders**)

Biliousness
Bile is a bitter, yellowish fluid secreted by the liver and stored in the gall bladder. It is discharged through the bile duct into the intestine where it assists in the process of digestion and assimilation. About a pint or more is secreted daily, but much of this is reabsorbed into the bloodstream and circulates back to the liver, to be again excreted, and so on. Biliousness is a rather vague term applied sometimes to migraine or to the sick headache and vomiting which occur in some forms of gastric catarrh or following indiscretions of diet. The liver salt, *Nat. Sulph.*, is the principal remedy indicated for disorders in the secretion and flow of bile. By irritating the epithelial cells and nerves of the bile ducts *Nat. Sulph.* helps the normal secretion of these organs, hence it is an excellent remedy for biliousness.

BIOCHEMIC TREATMENT
Nat. Sulph.   Symptoms arising from an excess of bile; bitter taste, vomiting of bile or bitter fluid, greenish stools. Greenish-brown coated tongue, yellow or sallow skin, yellow eyeballs.
Kali. Mur.   When associated with digestive orders with white-coated tongue or light-coloured stools.
Ferr. Phos.   For sick headache in alternation with *Nat. Sulph.*
See also Combination S.

Boils (see **Abscesses**)

Bones, Affections of
Various mineral salts are indispensable in the formation, growth and proper nourishment of the bone structure of the human body. *Calc. Phos.* prevents faulty growth and soft bones, and poor repair after fractures.
    Calc. Fluor. and *Silica* encourage the needed density to the outer surfaces and coverings of the bones.

BIOCHEMIC TREATMENT
Calc. Phos.   Weak soft bones in children. To promote the uniting of fractured bones.

Calc. Fluor. Disturbances on the surface of bones; hard, rough elevations. Bruises of the covering of bones.
Silica. Ulceration of the bones.

Bronchitis
Bronchitis is an inflammatory condition of the mucous membranes of the bronchial tubes. It may follow a cold or catarrh. The usual symptoms are feverishness with a harsh, dry cough and wheezing respiration. The painful chest symptoms become less distressing when expectoration begins. Rest in bed and a light diet, with warm drinks, are beneficial. If the inflammation spreads into the smaller bronchial tubes the symptoms become intensified with respiration rapid and difficult. Special care should be taken in the case of the very young and the aged.

BIOCHEMIC TREATMENT
Ferr. Phos. Is the first remedy for the inflammatory conditions, heat, fever and congestion. Short painful cough, without expectoration; short and oppressive breathing. *Ferr. Phos.* should be given in frequent doses in the acute stage, and when additional symptoms appear should be alternated with the remedy indicated by the expectoration, until all inflammatory symptoms disappear.
Kali. Mur. When the expectoration is thick, white, tenacious phlegm, and tongue has a white or greyish-white coating. Alternate with *Ferr. Phos.* when fever is present.
Kali Sulph. When the expectoration is light yellow, watery and copious, or greenish, slimy yellow. Alternate with *Ferr. Phos.* when fever is present to promote perspiration.
Silica. When the expectoration is thick, yellow and heavy; cough better after warm drink but aggravated by cold ones.
Nat. Mur. Bronchitis, with expectorations of clear, watery or frothy mucus. Alternate with *Ferr. Phos.* Chronic bronchitis, 'Winter cough', with watery symptoms. Phlegm is loose and rattling.
Calc. Phos. Expectoration of albuminous mucus (looks like white of egg before it is cooked, not watery). Bronchitis in anaemic persons, when the above symptoms are present.
See also Combination J.

Catarrh

An excessive secretion from the mucous membranes particularly those of the air passages. It usually begins as a nasal catarrh with a feeling of stuffiness and sneezing, accompanied by a profuse, watery discharge from the eyes and nose. Sometimes there is a loss of sense of smell and taste. There may also be soreness of the throat with bronchial irritation and symptoms similar to those of the common cold. The nature of the discharge is a guide to the tissue-salts required.

BIOCHEMIC TREATMENT

Ferr. Phos.   First or inflammatory stage. Catarrhal fever; congestion of nasal membranes.

Kali. Mur.   Second stage of catarrhal troubles, with white, thick, tenacious phlegm (not transparent). Catarrhs of the head, with stuffy sensations, white or grey-coated tongue; catarrh of any membrane, with a characteristic white bland discharge.

Nat. Mur.   Catarrhs with watery, transparent discharges. Catarrhs of anaemic people, with frothy discharges, sometimes having a salty taste. Catarrh of any membrane with above symptoms. Loss of sense of smell.

Calc. Phos.   Is an important remedy in catarrhal affections of anaemic persons and chronic cases. Should be given in all cases of catarrh, alternated with other indicated remedies, for its tonic action. Catarrh of any membrane, when the discharge is rich in albumin, transparent, like white of egg before it is cooked.

Kali. Sulph.   Third stage of all catarrhs, when the discharges or secretions are yellow, slimy or watery mucus. Thin, yellow discharge from the nose. Generally follows after *Kali. Mur.* Symptoms are worse in the evening or in a warm room.

Calc. Sulph.   Catarrh of any membrane, when the discharge is thick, yellow, watery, and sometimes mixed with blood.

Silica.   Chronic catarrh with offensive discharge. Excessive dryness or ulceration of the edge of the nostrils. Itching of the tip of the nose.

Calc. Fluor.   Stuffy catarrh of the head. Bronchial catarrh, when tiny, yellow, tough lumps of mucus are coughed up.

Nat. Sulph.   Catarrhs with profuse secretion of greenish mucus. Catarrhs of damp localities, aggravated at every change of the weather.

See also Combination Q.

Chilblains

An inflamed condition of the skin with swelling of the subcutaneous tissues, usually affecting the hands or feet. They occur in persons having a defective circulation and sometimes there is a nutritional deficiency. A nourishing diet and warm clothing are obvious preventive measures and regular exercise and massage, by helping to improve the circulation, remove the predisposing conditions.

BIOCHEMIC TREATMENT
Calc. Phos.   This is the principal remedy.
Kali. Mur.   Useful where there is much swelling.
Ferr. Phos.   In alternation with *Kali. Mur.* for the pain and inflammation.
Kali. Phos.   May be given intercurrently to counter the effects of the irritation.
Calc. Fluor.   A useful remedy when there are cracks in the skin.
Kali. Sulph.   Broken chilblains exuding thin, yellow fluid.
See also Combination P.

Colds

The so-called 'common cold' is an infectious disease caused by a virus, although there can be predisposing factors such as exposure to draughts, wetting of the feet etc. Some people are more likely to catch colds than others. A cold should never be neglected and if there is fever and congestion it is best to remain indoors. According to Dr Schuessler's System of Biochemistry, there is depletion of the mineral salts within the tissues of the respiratory tracts and especially the nose. A disturbed mineral salt balance may cause congestion of the tissues with uncombined albumin. This furnishes an ideal breeding ground for the bacteria which are the exciting cause of the inflammation.

Colds usually begin with a feeling of dryness and irritation in the nose, occasionally with smarting and burning and sneezing. This stage is quickly followed by a watery discharge from the nose, which may be bland or excoriating, and this in turn changes to a thick, yellowish discharge. Obstruction of the nose may accompany any or all stages of the disease. Chronic catarrh can follow.

BIOCHEMIC TREATMENT

Ferr. Phos.   Is needed for the feverishness, stuffiness and sneezing that herald the onset of a cold. That bout of sneezing is a first sign that a cold is threatening. It is a clear and unmistakable call for *Ferr. Phos.*

Kali. Mur.   For the second stage when there is white phlegm and stuffiness with congestion.

Nat. Mur.   Running, watery colds with chilliness and general feeling of discomfort. Loss of taste and smell and dryness of the skin.

Calc. Phos.   A short course of this remedy is helpful in building up the general health after a cold.

See also Combination J.

Colic

Colic is a pain due to irregular or violent contractions of muscular tissues in the body. The most usual form is that due to spasmodic contractions of the bowel and is called intestinal colic. There may be gastric colic in the stomach, biliary colic due to irregular contractions of the bile ducts, renal colic in the kidneys, etc. Infants are subject to attacks of colic, especially when fed artificially, and in such cases a modification of diet may be necessary.

BIOCHEMIC TREATMENT

Mag. Phos.   The remedy for pain, in alternation with the remedy indicated by the symptoms which gave rise to the pain. Colic of infants, with drawing up of the legs. Pain relieved by bending double. Flatulent colic, eased by friction, heat or belching gas. Colic coming and going by spells. Pains are crampy and constrictive, eased by heat.

Calc. Phos.   Should *Mag. Phos.*, though indicated, fail to give relief, *Calc. Phos.* is an alternative. Colic due to non-assimilation of food, or in teething children.

Nat. Phos.   Colic in children with acidity green sour-smelling stools.

Nat. Sulph.   Biliary colic, with vomiting of bile; bitter taste in the mouth and brownish-green coating on root of tongue.

Constipation

Though persons in health generally have one daily movement of the bowels, some may have two regular motions, while in others a motion once in two days is quite normal. When the bowel is evacuated too seldom or incompletely, the motions become dry and hard with difficulty of evacuation. There may be a mechanical obstruction of the bowel, but generally the condition is due to one or more of the following factors — too little 'roughage' in the diet, insufficient exercise, failure to inculcate the habit of regularity, dryness of the bowel, lack of tone of the colon muscle and of the villi of the intestines etc. The diet should include plenty of fresh fruit, green vegetables, green salads (uncooked), wholemeal bread and dried fruits such as prunes, which have an indigestible residue and thus provide bulk to exercise the intestinal muscles. Plenty of fluids, including raw fruit juices which provide water in its purest form. The regular use of aperients tends to aggravate the trouble.

BIOCHEMIC TREATMENT

Ferr. Phos.   Constipation, accompanied by a feeling of heat in the rectum, causing absorption of the natural fluids of the faeces and resulting in hardening and drying of the discharges. Piles, prolapus of the rectum, inflammations and fever are frequently associated with this type of constipation.

Kali. Mur.   Constipation, with light-coloured stools, from torpidity of the liver and want of bile. With white or greyish coated tongue, or when fat foods disagree.

Nat. Mur.   Constipation when caused from lack of moisture in the intestines. Dryness of the bowels, with watery secretions in other parts, watery eyes, excess of saliva, watery vomiting etc. Constipation with water-brash; dull heavy headache; hard, dry, black lumpy stools, difficult to pass; torn smarting feeling after stool.

Calc. Fluor.   Inability of muscles to expel faeces. The muscles of the rectum become relaxed, allowing a too large accumulation of faecal matter. Fissure of the anus, intensely sore crack near the lower margin.

Nat. Phos.   Constipation of infants, with occasional attacks of diarrhoea. Sore or acid conditions.

Nat. Sulph.   With bilious symptoms, hard, knotty stools; or soft stools difficult to expel.

Silica.   Faeces recede after having been partially expelled.

Convalescence

After an acute illness, the body requires a period of comparative rest in order to recuperate. Some acute ailments are attended by greater risks of a relapse during convalescence, and this applies particularly to those affecting respiration. During the period of recovery strenuous activities should be avoided and exposure to cold, damp, long hours of standing etc., reduced to a minimum.

BIOCHEMIC TREATMENT

Calc. Phos.   The principal remedy to restore the quality of the blood, to aid assimilation and tone up the system generally.

Kali. Phos.   Intercurrently to strengthen the nervous system.

Ferr. Phos.   In alternation with *Calc. Phos.* to oxygenize the blood. *See also Combination B.*

Coughs

Coughing is a symptom that occurs during the course of most diseases of the respiratory organs. It should not, however, be neglected as it may be the forerunner of more serious trouble, e.g. bronchitis, pneumonia etc. The nature and consistency of the expectoration point to the tissue-salt required. There are some coughs which are due to causes outside the respiratory tract and if there is no disease of this tract, medical advice should be sought.

BIOCHEMIC TREATMENT

Ferr. Phos.   First stage of all coughs. Short, acute, painful coughs, with soreness in the lungs and no expectoration. Tickling cough caused by irritation of the bronchial tubes. Hard and dry cough, with soreness of chest. For the inflammatory symptoms accompanying a cough.

Kali. Mur.   Loud, noisy and spasmodic coughs, accompanied with white or greyish-white coated tongue; the expectoration is thick, milky-white, tenacious. Croupy, hard cough; croup-like hoarseness.

Mag. Phos.   Paroxysms of coughing without expectoration. Spasmodic cough, loud and noisy, like whooping cough; relieved by hot drinks.

Kali. Sulph.   Late stage of inflammatory coughs, with expectoration of slimy, yellow or watery-yellow matter. Always worse in a warm room or in the evening; better in cool, open air. Hard, coarse croupy cough, with rattling of mucus in the chest.

Calc. Sulph.   Cough, when the expectoration is loose, mattery and sometimes streaked with blood.

Silica.   Chronic coughs, with thick, profuse, yellowish-green mattery expectoration; always worse in the morning on rising or on lying down at night; worse from cold drinks.

Nat. Mur.   Cough, with clear, watery expectoration, sometimes tasting salty, or with excessive discharge of watery secretions from the eyes, nose or mouth. In dry, tickling, hacking, irritating coughs.

Calc. Phos.   Expectoration clear but thick, rich in albumin — like the white of an egg before it is cooked. Intercurrently in all chronic coughs.

Nat. Sulph.   Cough with thick, ropy, greenish expectoration. Worse in damp weather. Soreness and pain in left chest; painful side when coughing.

Cramp

Is a painful spasmodic contraction of muscles, most frequently occurring in the limbs, but also apt to affect certain internal organs. This disorder belongs to the class of diseases known as local spasms, of which other varieties exist in such affections as spasmodic asthma and colic. The cause of these painful seizures resides in the nervous system, and operates either directly from the great nerve centres, or, as is generally the case, indirectly by reflex action, for example, when attacks are brought on by some derangement of the digestive organs.

BIOCHEMIC TREATMENT

Mag. Phos.   The principal remedy in cramps, spasms, neuralgias, twitchings, paroxysms, etc. Brings quicker relief when taken with a little hot water.

Calc. Phos.   In alternation with *Mag. Phos.* Sensation as if parts were asleep, and with feelings of numbness and cold.

Kali. Phos.   Intercurrently with *Mag. Phos.* and *Calc. Phos.*

Cystitis

Inflammation of the bladder is usually due to infection by a germ, together with a lowered state of health. Some types of germs are so powerful that they alone will cause inflammation of the bladder, but these are not common.

The causes which tend to lower the body's resistance are, injury or congestion of the bladder wall and stagnation of the urine.

Stagnation of the urine may be due to a variety of causes in the passage from the bladder to the exterior (the urethra), such as stricture (narrowing of the passage), enlargement of the prostate gland which surrounds the neck of the bladder, the presence of stone or other foreign body; and also various conditions affecting the nerve supply to the bladder.

Medical advice should be sought for cystitis.

EMERGENCY BIOCHEMIC TREATMENT

Ferr. Phos. First stage, frequent urination and burning pain. Difficult, suppressed with constant urging.

Kali. Mur. With swelling of the tissues, and thick white mucus in the urine. Urine dark red.

Kali. Phos. Cystitis when associated with nervousness, prostration. Scalding urination, cutting pain.

Mag. Phos. Ineffectual and painful straining, urine passes in drops. Severe spasmodic pains. Constant urging to urinate when standing or walking.

Diarrhoea

Diarrhoea is a symptom of many diseases and is one of the body's methods of ridding itself of unwanted substances. Diarrhoea in infants may be due to gastro-enteritis, a serious condition calling for prompt medical attention and careful nursing. A predisposing cause is artificial feeding; environment and seasonal factors should be taken into account.

Among the many causes of diarrhoea in adults are a catarrhal condition of the alimentary tract, emotional upsets, stomach chills, food poisoning, unwashed green-stuffs, unaccustomed foods and alcoholic drinks, particularly those indulged in during holidays overseas. Rest and warmth will give Nature a chance to deal with the trouble in her own way. A simple diet and the use of the appropriate tissue-salts will speed recovery.

BIOCHEMIC TREATMENT

Ferr. Phos. Diarrhoea of sudden onset, with fever, thirst. Diarrhoea caused by a chill; stools consist of undigested food, or watery, frequent stools.

Kali. Mur. Stools are light-coloured, pale yellow. White or slimy stools after eating rich food, with white coated tongue. Bloody or slimy stools.

Kali. Phos. Diarrhoea with foul-smelling stools; also when depression or exhaustion is present.

Kali. Sulph. Stools are yellow, watery and mattery; tongue coated light yellow; sometimes cramps in the bowels.

Nat. Mur. Stools are watery, caused by an excessive use of salt; stools cause soreness and smarting.

Nat. Sulph. Stools are dark or green, bilious. Chronic diarrhoea, with loose, watery, morning stools; worse in cold, wet weather. Diarrhoea of old people.

Nat. Phos. Stools are sour-smelling and green, due to acidity of the stomach and bowels. Summer diarrhoeas from eating unripe fruit, or associated with worms. Diarrhoeas of teething children with acid symptoms, and creamy, golden-yellow coating on the tongue.

Calc. Phos. One of the best remedies for diarrhoeas of teething children, due to poor assimilation of food; should be alternated with the remedy indicated by colour of the stool. Stools are hot, watery, offensive, profuse and sputtering; sometimes green or undigested. Diarrhoea in pale, anaemic children.

Mag. Phos. For cramp-like pain in the bowels, flatulent colic; relieved by hot applications. Alternate with the remedies indicated by colour of the stool.

Dysmenorrhoea (see **Female Disorders**)

Dyspepsia (see **Indigestion**)

Ear, Diseases of
Most of the diseases of the ear result from a secondary catarrhal infection, usually transmitted from the upper respiratory tract by means of the Eustachian tubes. Often the infection travels from the throat to the ear. Medical advice should always be sought for ear trouble.

BIOCHEMIC TREATMENT
Ferr. Phos. When inflammatory symptoms are present with fever,

pain, congestion, etc. Earache, with throbbing, burning pain; hot outward applications relieve. Noises in the ear from congestion. Temporary deafness, with cutting pain.

Kali. Mur. Secondary affections, after *Ferr. Phos.*, or in alternation with it. After inflammations — the membrane thickens causing deafness. Deafness, caused by swelling of the Eustachian tubes; also with swelling of the glands of the ear; cracking noises in the ear, when blowing the nose or on swallowing. Earache, with swelling of the glands or membranes of the throat or ear; tongue generally coated white; white catarrhal discharge from the ear.

Kali. Sulph. Earache, with thin, yellow, watery matter. Catarrh of the ear, with the above discharges; sharp pains under the ear. Tongue has a yellow slimy coating.

Silica. Foul, mattery discharges from the ear; *Silica* hastens suppuration.

Kali. Phos. Deafness, with noises in the ear; with weakness from nervous exhaustion.

Mag. Phos. Earache with sharp neuralgic pains in or around the ear.

Eyes, Diseases of

The delicacy of structure of the eye renders any disorder of this organ highly important. Many of its disorders cannot be cured or can be remedied only to a small extent, such, for example, as loss of transparency in the cornea; whilst, in the case of others, such as cataract and high errors of refraction, the skill of the specialist may restore the eye from a state of almost complete uselessness to that of good vision. Most of the diseases are intricate in their course and treatment, requiring the highest degree of skill and handling.

In the following account, some of the simpler eye disorders are dealt with. Defective vision and serious eye troubles should be treated by a physician, or an eye specialist.

BIOCHEMIC TREATMENT

Ferr. Phos. First stage of eye inflammation, for the redness, pain, etc. Burning in the eyes; pain in the eyeballs through overstraining the eyes; cold applications relieve. In granulated eyelids, for the pain and inflammation. Eyes bloodshot.

Kali. Mur. Second stage of inflammation, with discharge of white greyish-white matter. Sore eyes, with specks of white matter on lids. Granulated eyelids, with feeling of sand in the eyes. Alternate with *Ferr. Phos.*

Silica.   Inflammation, with thick, yellow discharges; styes on the eyelids; little boils and indurations around the eyelids.

Nat. Phos.   Inflammation, with discharges of golden-yellow, creamy matter, eyelids are stuck together in the morning; creamy coating on root of tongue.

Nat. Mur.   Eye affections, when there is a discharge of watery mucus or flow of tears; discharges cause soreness of the skin or the eruption of small blisters. Granulated eyelids, intercurrently with *Ferr. Phos.* and *Kali. Mur.*

Kali. Phos.   Neuralgic pains with flow of tears. Weak eyesight from weakness or exhaustion after disease.

Female Disorders

The Schuessler therapy is an excellent method of treatment of the various disorders peculiar to the female generative system. It rests upon the premise that the restoration of health is best accomplished through stimulation of the vital natural processes of the human system. The tissue-salts produce this with no untoward side-effects which can follow the use of drugs.

All the pelvic organs are lined with delicate mucous membranes, there are also many muscular and connective tissues and an abundance of nerve and blood vessels centred there: hence these parts are peculiarly susceptible to disturbing influences, apt to assume the form of one of the many disorders peculiar to women.

The very sensitive nature of these structures, however, makes them also quickly responsive to the beneficial healing influence of the tissue-salts.

Amenorrhoea (suppression of the menses)

Lessening of the menstrual flow may occur in varying degrees. It may be only a symptom of some disease, in which case the amenorrhoea will disappear when the disease is cured. Thus in anaemia of young girls, menstruation may become scanty, but will become normal again when the anaemia has been overcome.

Occasionally, women around thirty years of age who are overweight and unable to bear children, will have a premature cessation of menstruation, a condition which should come on about middle age. But the most commonly occurring and possibly most severe attacks of amenorrhoea, however, usually come on suddenly. These are generally caused by severe nervous shocks, exposure in cold or damp weather, and getting the feet wet, especially when this occurs near the time when menstruation is expected. In amenorrhoea appearing under such circumstances with nausea and headache also accompany the menstrual trouble.

BIOCHEMIC TREATMENT
Kali. Phos.   Suppression of flow with depressed spirits, lassitude and debility. Constant dull headaches, cross and irritable, fidgety.
Kali. Sulph.   Scanty or suppressed menses, with weight and fullness of abdomen.
Nat. Mur.   In young girls where menses do not appear, or when scanty and at long intervals.
Calc. Phos.   Amenorrhoea in anaemic patients.

Dysmenorrhoea (painful menstruation)
Dysmenorrhoea may be caused by lack of proper development of the uterus, by congestion and inflammation of the uterus and other pelvic organs or, rarely, by mechanical obstruction to the flow. In young girls the commonest cause is lack of proper nutrition, either of the pelvic organs alone or of the whole body.

Accompanying the nutritional disturbance there is usually some condition of the nervous system causing neuralgia.

In this form of dysmenorrhoea the patient seems normal until the approach of the menstrual period when neuralgic pains appear, increasing in severity until the flow is well established, when they subside. If the neuralgia effects the ovaries, the patient may suffer an attack of similar pain halfway between the periods.

Dysmenorrhoea caused by congestion or inflammation of the pelvic organs presents a different type of pain during menstruation. Here the sensation is that of soreness, heaviness and dull pain. The same symptoms are present during the interval between periods but not so severe.

BIOCHEMIC TREATMENT

Mag. Phos.   Is the chief remedy for the cramping, labourlike, bearing-down pains. Sharp cutting pain relieved by heat.

Ferr. Phos.   Painful menstruation, with bright red flow, flushed face and quickened pulse. Vomiting of undigested food. Congestion of the pelvic organs begins several days before the flow. Alternate with *Mag. Phos.* during the attack.

Kali. Phos.   Menstrual colic in pale, tearful, irritable, sensitive women; weakness of the nervous system, flow deep, dark red. Alternate with *Ferr. Phos.*

Calc. Phos.   Intercurrently in anaemic patients. In girls at puberty, scanty flow.

Kali. Mur.   When caused by taking cold; blood dark, blackish-red.

Nat. Mur.   Menses scanty and dark, preceded by frontal headache. Flow is irritating. Great mental depression.

Silica.   Icy coldness of the entire body before and during menses, with constipation and sweating of the feet.

See also Combination N.

Leucorrhoea (whites)

Leucorrhoea is caused by the secretion of an abnormal quantity of mucus in the mucous membrane which lines the vagina and uterus. This mucus is discharged from the body through the vagina, and may vary in colour from a thin, colourless fluid, like water, to a thick, milky-white fluid, sometimes tinged with blood.

    Leucorrhoea occurs most frequently in young, unmarried girls, in women after childbirth, and also in older women after the change of life. This is due to systemic weakness in young girls and mothers, and to changes which take place in the mucous lining of the vagina in older women.

    Other causes, however, such as taking cold, physical or nervous strain, etc., may also bring it on. Such cases are usually easier to cure than the ones mentioned in the preceding paragraph. But in any event, the basic cause of the leucorrhoea should be discovered as soon as possible, and efforts made to overcome it.

BIOCHEMIC TREATMENT

Kali. Mur.   Discharge of milky-white, non-irritating mucus, mild, profuse. Excellent in long standing cases.

Kali. Phos.   Leucorrhoea, scalding and acrid, yellowish, blistering, orange coloured.

Kali. Sulph.   Leucorrhoea, discharge of yellow, greenish, slimy or watery secretions.

Nat. Mur.   Leucorrhoea, a watery, scalding, irritating discharge, smarting after or between the periods.

Nat. Phos.   Leucorrhoea, discharge creamy or honey-coloured, or acrid, discharge from the uterus sour-smelling.

Nat. Sulph.   Leucorrhoea, acrid, corrosive.

Calc. Phos.   Leucorrhoea, as a constitutional tonic and intercurrent with the chief remedy; a discharge of albuminous mucus. Leucorrhoea worse after menses, looks like white of an egg.

Menopause (change of life)

The period of a woman's life during which the menses cease can be a critical time and care must be taken that harm is not done, particularly to the nervous system.

The onset of the change of life is usually gradual beginning around the forty-fifth year and continuing from one to three years and is marked by irregularity in the appearance of menstruation gradual diminution in the flow and by nervous manifestations.

Mental unrest is marked and there are frequent disturbances of the circulation, resulting in the hot flushes and chilly periods so common in this state.

Often the flow is profuse, especially following one or more missed periods, or may be irregularly scanty and profuse.

The digestive tract is frequently disturbed and indigestion is common.

BIOCHEMIC TREATMENT

Ferr. Phos.   Hot Flushes. Alternate with *Kali. Sulph.*

Kali. Phos.   Nervousness, mental depression, irritability, anxiety, fainting spells.

Calc. Phos.   General weakness, run-down condition, anaemia, loss of weight.

Menorrhagia (profuse menstruation)

This may be brought about by increased congestion of the pelvic organs. Simple anaemia may be a contributory cause in some cases.

BIOCHEMIC TREATMENT

Ferr. Phos.   Menses too frequent and too profuse, painful, blood bright red, congestion.

Kali. Mur.   Black, dark, clotted blood, catarrhal conditions.

Calc. Fluor.   Menorrhagia with bearing-down pains.

Calc. Phos.   Menses too early in young girls, also women when amaemia is present.

Pregnancy

During pregnancy a woman is required to carry on the process of life in her own body and, in addition, to provide all the material and life building processes for the formation and development of a new life. This places an added physiological demand on her. Added to this is the stress of modern life, with its influence upon the nervous system. A regular course of treatment with the tissue-salts, especially *Kali. Phos.* and *Calc. Phos.* for from three to six months preceding childbirth, will prove highly beneficial for both mother and child.

BIOCHEMIC TREATMENT

Kali. Phos.   During the period of pregnancy, especially if there is evidence of nervous strain.

Ferr. Phos.   Morning sickness during pregnancy, vomiting of undigested food.

Calc. Phos.   A valuable remedy during pregnancy, to aid normal development of the child. Weakness, weariness of the mother during and after pregnancy, poor assimilation of food.

Nat. Mur.   Morning sickness with frothy, watery phlegm.

Nat. Phos.   Morning sickness with vomiting of sour mucus, acidity of the stomach.

Nat. Sulph.   Vomiting of bilious matter, bitter taste.

Puberty

This is the age the girl develops into a woman and when menstruation first makes its appearance. Many girls pass through this stage of life without evidence of systemic disorders while others are troubled with nervous or mental disturbances.

BIOCHEMIC TREATMENT
Kali. Phos.   To tone up the nervous system.
Calc. Phos.   To improve nutrition.

Fever

Fever is a condition characterized by an increase in body temperature. It is one of the most common symptoms of disease but should be regarded as secondary to the disordered state with which it is associated. The temperature of the human body in health, ranges between 98.4 degrees and 99.5 degrees Fahrenheit. There are daily variations, the lowest being between the hours of midnight and 6 a.m. and the highest during the evening. The body normally maintains an even temperature by controlling the balance between heat gained and lost. Heat is gained by oxidation of the tissues, which takes place during the process of nutrition. Cooling occurs principally through the lungs and skin. In the feverish state balance is no longer maintained, more heat being lost than gained. A fever is usually preceded by chilliness and there may be headache or a feeling of tiredness in the limbs. There follows a 'hot' stage, the skin feels dry, there is an increase in the rate of the pulse, excessive thirst, and a little desire for food. Then follows some form of discharge, usually a profuse perspiration, after which the fever declines. In some diseases the fever may be continued or remittent.

BIOCHEMIC TREATMENT
Ferr. Phos.   The first remedy indicated in all types of fever. Rapid pulse, flushed face, sometimes accompanied by chilly sensation, vomiting of undigested food. *Ferr. Phos.* should be continued as long as the fever lasts, and alternated with such other tissue-salts as the subsequent symptoms indicate.
Kali. Mur.   Second stage of fevers, tongue covered with greyish-white coating. There is usually constipation present with light-coloured stools.
Kali. Sulph.   Evening rise of temperature with hot, dry skin; to promote perspiration.

Nat. Mur.   Early stages, excessive thirst, water does not relieve thirst; dry skin.

Fibrositis

Fibrositis is the popular term applied to muscular rheumatism. The onset may be acute or gradual. It can affect a whole area, such as back and shoulders, or be localized in one place. Exposure to damp and cold is a predisposing factor.

BIOCHEMIC TREATMENT
Ferr. Phos.   The principal remedy for acute, inflammatory pains brought on suddenly by chills, exposure, unaccustomed exercise, strains, etc.
Kali. Sulph.   When the pains are fleeting or shifting.
Mag. Phos.   Acute sharp spasmodic pains, relieved by warmth.
See also Combination I.

Gastric Disturbances

Gastric disturbances include a wide range of ailments characterized by painful or uncomfortable symptoms associated with the function of digestion. The symptoms are numerous and may arise from simple causes such as too hurried meals and insufficient mastication of the food. Diet is obviously important and the digestive organs should be given as much rest as possible by adopting regular habits and by the selection of wholesome, easily digestible foods. Acid dyspepsia, catarrh of the stomach and nervous dyspepsia are some of the conditions that come under this general heading.

BIOCHEMIC TREATMENT
Ferr. Phos.   Gastritis and pain, swelling, and tenderness of the stomach. Dyspepsia with hot, flushed face. Vomiting of undigested food, the tongue being clean.
Kali. Mur.   Gastric derangements when the tongue has a white or greyish-white coating. Indigestion or nausea after taking fatty or rich foods. In alternation with *Ferr. Phos.* in the treatment of gastritis.
Nat. Phos.   Gastric derangements with symptoms of acidity. Sour risings, creamy, golden-yellow coating on the back part of the tongue. Heartburn after eating. Fretful, irritable disposition.

Calc. Phos.   A useful remedy in the treatment of gastric and digestive disturbances when taken in alternation with other indicated remedies. It aids the digestive processes and improves assimilation.

Kali. Phos.   Nervous indigestion with 'gone' sensation in the stomach. Hungry feeling after taking food. Stomach-ache after fright or from excitement.

Kali. Sulph.   Gastric catarrh with slimy golden-yellow coating of the tongue. Colicky pains in the stomach with feeling of pressure or fullness.

Mag. Phos.   Spasmodic pains and cramp of the stomach, relieved by hot drinks. Flatulence with much belching of gas.

Nat. Sulph.   Gastric disturbances with bilious symptoms, bitter taste in the mouth, vomiting of bitter fluids. The tongue is sometimes coated a greenish-brown or greenish-grey colour.

See also Combinations C and S.

Gout

Gout is a constitutional disease in which there is an excess of uric acid in the blood. It has a marked tendency to be hereditary and it could be regarded as a good example of a disease in which the children suffer for the medical sins of their fathers. Those who come from 'gouty stock' may become typically gouty in their old age. Those who lead a sedentary life and indulge in rich food and liquor appear to be predisposed to this disease.

Gout is more common in mature age than in the earlier years of life. In a typical attack of gout there is a severe pain in a joint, usually the big toe. The joint swells and becomes intensely hot. Any jarring of the affected joint causes extreme pain. When the trouble assumes a chronic form, the joint becomes permanently enlarged and remains tender and sensitive at all times.

BIOCHEMIC TREATMENT

Ferr. Phos.   For the fever and other inflammatory symptoms.

Nat. Sulph.   The chief remedy in this affection, especially if due to rich food, or when there are bilious symptoms present. In acute attacks alternate with *Ferr. Phos.*

Nat. Phos.   If acid conditions are in evidence, cream coated tongue, sour-smelling sweat, etc. Chronic Gout.

Haemorrhoids

Haemorrhoids (piles) are a varicosed condition of the veins at the lower end of the bowel. Piles may be internal or external, or both. Internal piles extend about one inch up the bowel. Sedentary habits are a predisposing factor and constipation with straining at stool is not an unusual accompaniment of this painful condition. Piles sometimes occur during pregnancy and they can also be a symptom of other diseases. External piles need not necessarily cause any pain or trouble. Sometimes they may become inflamed and give off a thin discharge. Internal piles may give no sign of their presence except for occasional bleeding. Too great a loss of blood will cause anaemia. When internal piles are large they may protrude and become inflamed and painful. In general piles are more of an inconvenience than a serious condition. Care should be taken to avoid constipation and it is better to achieve this by regulating the diet than by recourse to purgatives, which in the long run aggravate the trouble. The parts should be carefully washed after evacuation and any protrusions gently replaced. Piles tend to be one of the ailments of middle age.

BIOCHEMIC TREATMENT

Ferr. Phos.   For the inflammation and bleeding.

Calc. Fluor.   Internal and blind piles, sometimes accompanied by pain in the back. Tones up the relaxed condition of the veins and muscular fibres.

Calc. Phos.   Intercurrently with *Calc. Fluor.* in anaemic people.

See also Combination G.

Hair, Falling Out of

Everyday, in the healthy scalp, a certain number of hairs reach the end of their existence, and fall out, being replaced in time by new hairs. Each follicle produces many hairs in the course of a lifetime, but sometimes the hairs gradually become finer and the hair producing quality of the follicle finally fails. This may be due to an eczematous condition of the scalp, or dandruff, and to a certain extent, it may be hereditary. Some diseases may cause partial loss of hair and prolonged anxiety or nervous shock are known to be responsible.

BIOCHEMIC TREATMENT
Kali. Sulph.   Falling-out hair, bald spots. Much scaling of the scalp, moist and sticky. Dandruff.
Silica.   Impoverished condition of the hair, lack lustre. A valuable hair conditioner.
Nat. Mur.   A useful supplementary remedy in cases of dandruff and falling-out hair.
Kali. Phos.   Loss of hair when due to nervous causes.
Calc. Phos.   Loss of hair when due to defective nutrition.
See also Combination K.

Hay Fever

Hay fever is an allergic condition of the mucous membranes of the eyes, nose and air passages. One of the predisposing factors is hereditary. It is twice as common in men as women and it seems to affect those of active temperament and high mental development. Attacks of hay fever can be brought on from pollen, spores and fungi. The eyes and nose are most commonly involved, the bronchi frequently, when the disease is called pollen-asthma. The attack commences with irritation of the nasal membrane, swelling, dryness and tickling culminating in sneezing, quickly followed by a profuse watery discharge from the nose and usually from the eyes at the same time. There is smarting and burning of both the nose and eyes. This is the common type, although many develop symptoms of bronchial origin and some have typical attacks of asthma. It is suggested that those who are annually troubled with hay fever should use the indicated tissue-salts approximately four to six weeks prior to the expected attack of hay fever, and continue the treatment during the actual hay fever season.

BIOCHEMIC TREATMENT
Nat. Mur.   For hay fever after exposure to sun; watery symptoms with sensation of itching and tingling in the nose.
Mag. Phos.   To prevent a threatened attack from maturing, or to relax the spasms.
Silica.   Itching and tingling of the nose with violent sneezing.
Kali. Phos.   For the depression and to aid breathing.
Ferr. Phos.   For the congestion, inflammation and headache.
See also Combination H.

Headache

Headache is one of the most commonplace of human ailments. It is symptomatic of many diseased conditions, some slight and others more serious, and it can arise from a variety of causes. The brain itself is insensitive to pain. It is probable that the pain of headache is due to dilatation, a response to nervous stimuli, or the pain may arise from the neck muscles, or scalp, or from other nearby organs. One of the most frequent causes of headache is anxiety and living at too high a pressure.

Defective eyesight is another common cause. The pain occurs in the region of the brow and tends to come on in the evening, particularly if a lot of reading or close work has been done during the day. Sinus infection is less a common cause and in such cases there is usually a history of colds in the head. Septic teeth can also be responsible for headaches.

Constipation is a common cause, especially in children. Headaches are also a characteristic feature of fevers.

These are some of the factors responsible for headaches and in treating the trouble it is necessary to search out and remove the cause. Although the pain-killing drugs have their place, their continued use to suppress symptoms is not advisable and some could result in harmful side-effects, e.g. stomach haemorrhage.

BIOCHEMIC TREATMENT

Ferr. Phos.   Headaches of an inflammatory nature, with bruising, pressing, stitching pains; congestive headaches, red face or blood-shot eyes, throbbing headache, in the temples or over the eyes; blinding, sick headaches, with vomiting of undigested food. Scalp sore or tender to the touch; headaches from excessive heat or cold. Congestive headache at the menstrual period. Alternate with the remedy indicated by the colour of the tongue. All pains worse from motion and noise.

Kali. Phos.   Headaches of purely nervous character, resulting from overstrain of the mental faculties, worry, sleeplessness, etc. Headaches of nervous, sensitive, pale, irritable or excitable persons. Students' headaches; headaches with inability for thought, better under cheerful excitement, or with gentle motion; tongue is frequently coated like stale mustard; bad breath.

Kali. Mur.   With sluggish action of the liver, white-coated tongue or vomiting and hawking of milk-white mucus.

Nat. Mur.   Dull, heavy headache, with profusion of tears, watery discharge from the nose, or excessive flow of saliva; frequently associated with constipation of the bowels. Headaches with sleepiness, unrefreshing sleep. Vomiting of watery transparent fluids.

Headaches of young girls with irregular menstruation, with watery symptoms. Pains are generally worse in the morning and disappear in the evening.

Mag. Phos.   Neuralgic headaches, pains are excruciating, stinging, shooting, darting, intermittent or in paroxysms. Heat relieves, cold aggravates; headaches with 'sparks' before the eyes. Nervous headaches, with cramp pains, worse from cold draughts of air.

Nat. Sulph.   Bilious headaches; vomiting of bile, bitter taste, greenish-grey coated tongue, colic pains or bilious diarrhoea. Sick headaches, with giddiness, vertigo, and dullness. Violent pains at the base of the brain or on the top of the head; cannot tolerate noise.

Nat. Phos.   Headaches on the crown of the head, with acid conditions; on awakening in the morning; with acid, sour risings; vomiting of sour or acid fluids. The tongue generally has a creamy, moist yellow coating on the back part or in the roof of the mouth.

Calc. Phos.   Headaches, with cold feelings in the head, or with creeping coldness and numbness on the head. Pains are worse from heat or cold. Neuralgic headache should *Mag. Phos.* fail to relieve.

Calc. Sulph.   Headache with vertigo and nausea. Pain around the whole head.

See also Combinations F and S.

Hiccups

Hiccups is a spasmodic contraction of the muscles of the diaphragm closing the throat, resulting in a sudden shutting off of breath. It is brought about by an irritation of the nerves which serve the diaphragm, usually following some digestive upset.

BIOCHEMIC TREATMENT

Mag. Phos.   The principal remedy. It should be given with a little hot water.

Nat. Phos.   In alternation with *Mag. Phos.* if the spasms persist.

Hives (Nettle-rash or Urticaria)

Hives is a disorder of the skin characterized by an eruption resembling the effect produced by the sting of a nettle, namely, raised red or red-and-white patches, occurring in parts or over the whole of the surface of the body, and attended with great itching and irritation.

In many cases the attack appears to be connected with digestive derangements, or the taking of certain articles of diet particularly of protein nature, such as various kinds of meat, fish, shell-fish etc., also occasionally from the use of certain drugs.

BIOCHEMIC TREATMENT
Ferr. Phos.   When there is feverishness.
Kali. Sulph.   When the skin is dry and tending to scale.
Nat. Mur.   Eruptions with clear, watery, contents, nettle-rash after becoming overheated.
Nat. Phos.   Soreness of the skin, with symptoms of acidity. Creamy exudations.

Hoarseness

Hoarseness or huskiness of the voice is generally the result of catarrh or inflammation of the vocal cords, but it may also result from pressure on the nerves that control the movements of the cords. Disease in the region of the glottis will affect the voice, or sore throat may arise from over-use of the voice and cause a certain amount of hoarseness.

BIOCHEMIC TREATMENT
Ferr. Phos.   Painful hoarseness of speakers and singers, with inflammation; from over-exertion of the voice, or from catching cold.
Kali. Mur.   Hoarseness, huskiness from cold. Second stage, loss of voice.
Kali. Phos.   If there is exhaustion, tired weary feeling in the throat.
Calc. Phos.   When the phlegm is albuminous (like white of an egg); alternate with *Ferr. Phos.*

Indigestion (see Gastric Disturbances)

Influenza

Influenza is one of the infectious, febrile diseases principally involving the respiratory organs. It occurs usually in epidemics during the winter months. The Italians at one time ascribed it to the influence of the stars, hence the name 'influenza'. It is now known to be due to a virus. The onset of influenza is sudden with a feeling of chilliness, headache and aching of the limbs, followed by sore throat and other symptoms. Old people, particularly, are susceptible to complications. Heart symptoms are common and constitute one of the major dangers of influenza. Inflammation of the middle ear is not uncommon following influenza, an aftermath is depression, which may even amount to melancholia. Extra care should be taken during convalescence to avoid the possibility of a relapse.

BIOCHEMIC TREATMENT

Ferr. Phos.   In the first stage with chills, followed by heat, fever, headache, vomiting.

Nat. Sulph.   The principal remedy to eliminate the excess of toxic fluids resulting from infection.

Kali. Sulph.   In alternation with *Ferr. Phos.* to promote perspiration. Dry skin, feeling of heat.

Kali. Mur.   Sore throat, the tongue has a white-coated appearance.

Nat. Mur.   For the watery conditions, tears, running from the nose, sneezing, dry throat, etc.

Calc. Phos.   Weakness and physical lassitude during and after convalescence.

Jaundice

Jaundice is due to the presence of bile in the blood which causes the skin to turn yellowish in colour. There are many different causes of this condition, and naturally the symptoms vary in accordance with the cause. The commonest form is that known as catarrhal jaundice, due to an inflammation or catarrh of the bile-duct which prevents the flow of bile from the liver and gall-bladder into the intestine. This inflammation, it has been found, usually begins in the duodenum, or first part of the small intestine, then spreads to the bile-duct where it causes an obstruction.

BIOCHEMIC TREATMENT

Ferr. Phos.   Early stage, inflammatory condition, fever, pain in liver, vomiting of undigested food.

Nat. Sulph.   Congestion of the liver and gall-bladder with resulting jaundice. Biliousness, flatulence, cutting pains, greenish stools.
Kali. Mur.   Jaundice with catarrhal condition. Constipation, light coloured stools; white-coated tongue, bitter taste. Vomiting of thick white mucus.
Nat. Mur.   Jaundice associated with catarrh of the stomach, drowsiness, watery secretions, thirst, dryness of the skin.

Laryngitis
Acute laryngitis usually begins with a cold and it may be accompanied by severe pain deep in the throat.
   Chronic laryngitis is usually caused by strain, often seen in singers, clergymen and school teachers. An essential in treating chronic laryngitis is to rest the voice.

BIOCHEMIC TREATMENT
Ferr. Phos.   Painful hoarseness of speakers and singers due to strain on the vocal cords or from catching cold; soreness of the larynx, fever.
Kali. Mur.   Loss of voice from cold. Croupy cough with expectoration of thick, white, tenacious mucus. Tongue white.
Kali. Phos.   Hoarseness after nervous strain; tired, weary feeling, general weakness.
Calc. Phos.   Chronic hoarseness, with much hemming and scraping of the throat.

Lumbago
Lumbago is a form of rheumatism affecting the muscles of the lower part of the back. It is sometimes brought on by exposure to cold and damp or unaccustomed exercise, such as bending and lifting. There is an inflammatory condition of the muscular tissues (*Ferr. Phos.*) with congestion and pressure upon the nerve endings. Lumbago usually comes on suddenly, like a stab in the back, and it may be difficult or impossible to move on account of the pain. The attacks are usually of short duration. Treatment is on similar lines to that recommended for rheumatism. The local application of heat and gentle massage, if this can be borne, should bring a measure of relief.

BIOCHEMIC TREATMENT
Ferr. Phos.   Early stage, fever, inflammation, severe pain.
Nat. Phos.   Lumbago with acid condition; sour, acid perspiration; rheumatic tendency.
Calc. Phos.   Backache and stiffness from slightest draught, worse in the morning.
Calc. Fluor.   Lumbago following a strain.
Nat. Mur.   Lumbago relieved by lying on something hard. Pain as if bruised from prolonged stooping. Sensation of coldness up and down the spine.
See also Combination G.

Nervous Debility

This is a state where nerve force is being used up more quickly than it can be generated, and when we recognize this simple fact we realize that to stimulate the nerves with so-called 'tonics' is one way of aggravating the trouble. Grief, worry, undue mental exertion, irregular habits, emotional extravagance; these are the parasitical influences which rob the nerves of their vitality. Treatment should aim to increase the supply of nervous energy and to bring the nerves back to a state of normal tranquillity. When this has been achieved a remarkable change for the better will be experienced.

BIOCHEMIC TREATMENT
Kali. Phos.   This is the principal nerve tissue-salt; the nerve vitaliser which should be given in ailments of a nervous character. It is the remedy when the nerves are said to be 'on edge'.
Mag. Phos.   This tissue-salt acts well with *Kali. Phos.* but has more to do with the motor nerves. *Mag. Phos.* is indicated for nerve pains, cramps and nervous twitchings. It helps to steady the nerves.
Calc. Phos.   This tissue-salt is needed to raise the general nutritional tone and to improve the quality of the blood. It promotes the assimilation of vital nutrients and so contributes to the supply of nervous energy. Other tissue-salts may be needed to deal with individual symptoms but the above are the most frequently needed remedies for ailments of a truly nervous character.
See also Combination B and 'Nervone'.

Neuralgia

Neuralgia is pain felt along a nerve. There are very many different causes of neuralgia as well as many different positions where the pain may be felt, but the character of the pain is nearly always the same. The pain of neuralgia is of a severe shooting or throbbing nature and the skin, along which tiny branches of the nerves run, is often very tender to touch. Another curious feature of the pain of neuralgia is that it is not continuous but occurs in little bouts, which are made worse by exposing the skin to the cold. Neuralgia may be the result of changes in the nerves, when the pain is said to be due to neuritis; or the nerves themselves may be perfectly healthy, the pain being caused by pressure on the nerves by other structures; or the nerves may be irritated by some disease of structures with which they are in contact.

BIOCHEMIC TREATMENT

Mag. Phos. The chief remedy for all neuralgic pains; intense, darting, excruciating, or spasmodic pains; pains relieved by heat and aggravated by cold. This tissue-salt will act more rapidly when taken with a little warm water.

Kali. Phos. Neuralgic pains in nervous, sensitive persons. Pains are better after gentle motion. Pains with depression; failure of strength, nervousness, sleeplessness, irritability, crossness, etc. Feeling of numbness.

Nat. Mur. Severe neuralgic pains, intermittent and with excessive flow of saliva or tears. The pains resemble those of *Mag. Phos.*, but are distinguished from them by the excessive secretions of fluids from the mucous membrane of some organ.

Ferr. Phos. Neuralgic pains due to inflammatory conditions, caused by a chill or cold; severe throbbing pains, like a nail being driven in over the eye; blinding pains, with a fever, burning heat, flushed face.

Calc. Phos. Pains coming on at night and of a numbing character, or with sensation of crawling or coldness; deep-seated pains; neuralgia in anaemic persons.

Nat. Sulph. Neuralgia brought on by damp weather or living in damp house.

Silica. Neuralgic pain in the teeth.

Calc. Sulph. This remedy occupies a ground between the very acute

pains of *Mag. Phos.* and the paralysing ones of *Kali. Phos.* (more in aged persons, if there be a want of regenerative force for the nervous tissue).
See also Combination A and 'Nervone'.

Neuritis
Neuritis means inflammation affecting a nerve or nerves which may be localized to one part of the body, as, for instance, in sciatica, facial neuralgia due to this cause, etc., or which may be general, being then known as 'multiple neuritis'.

BIOCHEMIC TREATMENT
Ferr. Phos.   Early stage, congestive and inflammatory condition, severe pain, fever. Neuritis from exposure to cold.
Kali. Phos.   Sharp pains, worse at rest and when beginning to move; difficulty in moving the limbs.
Mag. Phos.   Severe, acute pains, failing strength in muscles.
See also Combination A.

Piles (see Haemorrhoids)

Prostatic Disorders
The prostate gland is a structure which lies at the neck of the bladder in men and surrounds that part of the urethra lying within the pelvis. This gland is of importance because in late life it is apt to increase in size and change in shape in such a way as to obstruct the exit of urine from the bladder.

   In the large majority of cases in which enlargement of the prostate gland produces such an obstruction, removal by means of operation is recommended.

BIOCHEMIC TREATMENT
Ferr. Phos.   Acute prostatic congestion, irritation, retention of urine, or difficult urination. Fever.
Calc. Fluor.   Enlargement of the prostate gland.
Nat. Sulph.   A useful intercurrent remedy.

Rheumatism

A collective term covering a variety of conditions involving inflammation of the connective tissues of muscles and joints and characterized by pain in the affected parts. There are several factors, some or all of which may be concerned in the cause of rheumatism, such as, focal infection, acidity, heredity, toxaemia, and exposure to inclement weather.

At the onset there is a measure of congestion and inflammation and if this can be broken up promptly a serious attack may be averted. For this purpose the tissue-salt *Ferr. Phos.* is needed. *Ferr. Phos.* is useful as a first-aid for accute attacks of rheumatism.

Another associated symptom of rheumatism is acidity. Faulty elimination allows the accumulation in the blood of acid-waste products which have a bad effect on the general circulation. The acid-neutralizing tissue-salt, *Nat. Phos.*, breaks up these harmful acids and so helps to bring about their elimination.

In rheumatic ailments, all the eliminative organs are involved. Kidneys, liver, bowels, lungs — even the skin. There is some hold-up in the body's waste transport system, the organs concerned are lacking in tone and efficiency. The great vitalizer of this transport system is *Nat. Sulph.* This tissue-salt brings about the removal of the poison charged fluids which are the normal result of the chemical exchanges constantly taking place in the living tissue-cells. If conditions arise which allow these waste matters to accumulate in the blood and tissues, then self poisoning results. The importance of *Nat. Sulph.* to rheumatic subjects thus becomes self-evident.

Other tissue-salts may sometimes be required owing to complication conditions, but the three tissue-salts mentioned are the ones most frequently needed.

BIOCHEMIC TREATMENT

Ferr. Phos.   In the first stages of rheumatism, for the pain, fever, heat, redness, quickened pulse. Rheumatism located in any part; fibrositis, pains are increased by movement; soreness and stiffness all over the body. Growing pains of children.

Kali. Mur.   Second stage of rheumatism or fibrositis, when swelling has resulted (alternate with *Ferr. Phos.*). Tongue with thick, white or greyish coating. Swelling of the joints. Movement increases the pains.

Nat. Phos.   One of the principal remedies. Sour-smelling perspiration or acid conditions; acid taste in the mouth; creamy-yellow coating on the base of the tongue.

Nat. Sulph.   To aid in removing toxic-charged fluids from the system.

Silica.   To break up accumulation of urates lodging around the joints and muscles.

Calc. Phos.   Rheumatism which is worse at night and in bad weather, heat or cold, dampness, and change of weather. Stiffness and numbness of the joints.

Calc. Fluor.   Enlargement of the joints from rheumatism.

Mag. Phos.   Acute, sharp spasmodic pains in rheumatism; excruciating, violent pains relieved by warmth.

See also Combination M and Zief.

Sciatica

Sciatica is inflammation of the great sciatic nerve which runs down the back of the thigh. It can follow as a result of exposure to cold and damp, causing irritation of the nerve. There may be a rheumatic tendency. Pressure from other causes may also be responsible for sciatic pain. A slipped vertebral disc is not an uncommon cause of pain in the sciatic nerve. The trouble may first be felt a little behind the hip joint, and then extending downwards even as far as the foot. Hip, knee and ankle joints are particularly tender areas. In severe cases movement of the limb is very painful and rest in bed becomes necessary.

BIOCHEMIC TREATMENT

Ferr. Phos.   For the general pain and inflammation.

Mag. Phos.   When the pain is spasmodic.

Kali. Phos.   In alternation with *Mag. Phos.* when there is nervous exhaustion with great restlessness.

Nat. Sulph.   Pain when getting up from sitting or turning in bed, no relief in any position.

See also Combination A.

Sinus

Sinus is a cavity in bone or tissue. The air sinuses of the frontal bones communicate with the interior of the nose. Inflammation or infection may spread into the sinus cavities and may be difficult to disperse on account of the restricted drainage apertures. Suppuration into the nasal sinuses may be associated with an abscess of the upper teeth, the roots of which project into the cavity. Nasal catarrh may also spread into the sinus.

BIOCHEMIC TREATMENT

Ferr. Phos.　First stage, fever and congestion and pain in the sinus area. Flushed face, rapid pulse, throbbing pain.

Kali. Mur.　Dull pain in the sinus area, thick white mucus discharge, stuffiness of the head.

Nat. Mur.　Nasal obstruction with watery discharge, loss of sense of smell, inflammation of sinus with sensation of beating as of hammers, worse in cold air.

Kali. Sulph.　Yellow, slimy discharges, worse in warm room and in evening.

Silica.　Chronic condition; thick, offensive, acrid discharge, ulceration of mucous membrane, chronic nasal catarrh.

See also Combination Q.

Skin Ailments

Skin ailments are a large and important group which not only influence the general health, but may reveal constitutional weaknesses both inherited and acquired. There are several broad classifications, those affecting the sebaceous and sweat glands, inflammatory diseases, nervous disorders, and those due to parasitic infections.

It should be borne in mind that the skin is an important organ of elimination and that most forms of discharge are indications that the system is throwing-off unwanted organic materials which for some reason have become non-functional. Seborrhoea is a term applied to an accumulation of sebaceous secretions forming scales mostly on the scalp and which may interfere with the growth of the hair. Acne is a somewhat similar form of eruption occurring more on the face and upper part of the body, and especially during adolescence. Careful cleansing of the affected parts is necessary. A wart (verruca) is an excrescence from the surface of the skin, which sometimes disappears spontaneously or may have to be excised. Inflammatory affections are symptomatic of many fevers and may take various forms.

Nettle-rash is a diffuse redness of the skin accompanied by weals similar to the effect of stinging nettles.

'Catarrhal' conditions of the skin are a large and important group, the most common being eczema, which may be wet or dry. Shingles is a painful eruption which may attack any part of the body but always along the distribution of a nerve. Shingles is more frequently met with in elderly people and it can be a very debilitating ailment.

BIOCHEMIC TREATMENT

Ferr. Phos.   In the first stage of skin diseases, when there is fever, inflammation, heat, pain, burning etc.

Kali. Mur.   Second stage of inflammatory conditions. Eruptions on any part of the body or limbs, when the contents are thick and white; generally accompanied with a white-coated tongue, swelling of the affected parts. Warts, shingles in alternation with *Nat. Mur.*

Kali. Sulph.   All eruptions of the skin, when the discharges are watery, yellow and foul matter. Greenish-yellow exudate and the formation of crusts. Dry skin; sudden suppression of eruptions; peeling of the skin, with or without sticky secretions. Brittle nails in alternation with *Silica*. The principal tissue-salt for psoriasis and also athlete's foot.

Nat. Mur.   All affections with watery blisters and thin, transparent, white scales. Skin greasy, especially on the hairy parts. Skin and hair dry, hair falls out. Shingles where irritation is felt. Effects of insect bites; itching and burning of the skin. Skin affections accompanied by watery discharges which burn and irritate the parts. Eczema in bend of joints. Tongue clean but with frothy bubbles along the edge.

Nat. Phos.   All skin eruptions, when the discharges are creamy, golden-yellow or coloured like honey, irritating; symptoms of acidity and sour smelling perspiration; creamy-yellow coating on the root of the tongue.

Kali. Phos.   Eczema and eruptions of the skin, if accompanied with offensive odour; exhausting perspirations, nervousness; secretions cause soreness. Itching of chilblains. Pruritus in alternation with *Calc. Phos.*

Calc. Phos.   Skin affections, when the secretions consist of albuminous fluid (like the white of an egg before it is cooked). Skin diseases, when associated with anaemic conditions. Skin becomes red and itches after application of water. Pruritus in alternation with *Kali. Phos.*

Calc. Sulph. Discharge of thick, yellow matter with yellowish scabs; unhealthy wounds with pus which will not heal. Pimples, pustules occurring during adolescence.

Silica. To hasten suppuration. Secretions are mattery, or blood and matter. Offensive odour and sweating of the feet. Boils, ulcers with tendency to suppurate. Diseased and softened nails. Symptoms are worse from cold; better from warmth. In alternation with *Kali. Sulph.*

Nat. Sulph. Discharges are yellowish and watery; moist skin affections, with yellowish scabs or scales; chafing of the skin. Symptoms are generally associated with bilious conditions. Symptoms aggravated and accompanied by greenish-brown coating of the tongue and bitter taste.

Calc. Fluor. Chaps and cracks of the skin; cracks in palms of hands. Fissures about the nails, around the anus and mouth. Brittle finger nails, if *Kali. Sulph.* and *Silica* are non-effective. Thickening of the skin which becomes hard and tough.

See also Combination D.

Sleeplessness

Sleeplessness may be due to various causes. People of a highly-strung disposition find it more difficult to relax — nervous tension, aggravated by worry, anxiety, overwork, etc., is one of the more common factors. Indigestion is responsible in many cases and the eating of a heavy meal and stimulants too soon before retiring should be avoided. The brain sometimes becomes over-active as a result of late night work so that it is difficult to settle down to sleep. A certain amount of mental effort is called for to stem the kaleidoscope of thoughts that tend to crowd the mind. *Kali. Phos.* is helpful as a constitutional remedy when the nervous system is run-down. Elderly people usually need less sleep and sleeplessness at night can sometimes be made good by a 'nap' after lunch.

BIOCHEMIC TREATMENT

Kali. Phos. Sleeplessness following excitement, mental overwork, business troubles and from nervous causes generally.

Ferr. Phos. Sleeplessness, from feverish congestions. Drowsy in the afternoon but unable to sleep at night.

Nat. Mur. Excessive or constant desire to sleep; usual amount of sleep is unrefreshing; frequent starting during sleep which is restless.

Nat. Sulph.   Drowsiness or sleepiness, when the tongue has a greyish or brownish-green coating, bitter taste in the mouth, and when associated with bilious symptoms. Much dreaming soon after falling alseep.

Mag. Phos.   Sleeplessness, when the brain feels as if it is contracted, arising from nervous causes; spells of yawning.

Nat. Phos.   Sleeplessness due to digestive disturbances and when there are symptoms of acidity.

Sore Throat

An inflammatory condition of the wall of the throat (the pharynx) is known as pharyngitis and inflammation of the mucous membrane of the larynx (the organ of the voice) is laryngitis. The term 'throat' is popularly applied to the region about the front of the neck, but, correctly speaking, it means the irregular cavity into which the nose and mouth open above, and from which the larynx and gullet lead below, where the channel for the air and that for the food intersect.

Pharyngitis may be due to infection, digestive disturbances, too much smoking etc. and in severe cases there may even be slight bleeding of the smaller blood vessels. There is usually irritation, cough, and general discomfort. Laryngitis is brought on by similar causes including exposure to damp and draughts, too much talking, etc., and it is also a symptom of many infectious diseases. There may be swelling and difficulty in breathing. The heat, pain and dryness are a clear call for *Ferr. Phos.*, which should be given at frequent intervals during the acute stage until the inflammation subsides.

BIOCHEMIC TREATMENT

Ferr. Phos.   For the inflammation and burning pain. Throat red and dry with hoarseness, loss of voice.

Kali. Mur.   In alternation with *Ferr. Phos.* when there is swelling of the glands or tonsils.

Calc. Sulph.   If taken in the early stages can prevent development of a cold. In the later stages of tonsillitis when matter is discharged or abscess forms. Ulcerated sore throat.

Calc. Fluor.   Relaxed throat with tickling in the larynx. In alternation with *Calc. Phos.* for enlargement of the tonsils.

Calc. Phos.   Sore, aching throat with pain or swallowing. Chronic enlargement of tonsils.

Sunstroke

Sunstroke, more accurately called heatstroke, is a condition of the body produced by exposure to great heat, combined ordinarily with marked humidity of the atmosphere. Sun exposure is not necessary to bring on this trouble, as artificial heat will produce the same result. When the air is hot and moist, perspiration, which ordinarily by its evaporation cools the temperature of the body, does not evaporate but remains in drops upon the skin, while the body accumulates heat until temperature is so high that a heatstroke is brought on.

BIOCHEMIC TREATMENT
Nat. Mur.   This is the chief remedy to regulate the distribution of moisture. It should be given at frequent intervals.
Ferr. Phos.   In alternation with *Nat. Mur.* for the inflammatory symptoms and to help respiration.

Synovitis

Synovitis is inflammation of the membrane lining a joint. There is usually an effusion of fluid with swelling and pain. It occurs in certain rheumatic diseases and also as a result of injuries and strains, particularly those arising from athletic activities. Bursitis is a somewhat similar condition.

BIOCHEMIC TREATMENT
Ferr. Phos.   For the pain, stiffness and inflammation.
Nat. Sulph.   To disperse the infiltration of fluid.
Silica.   For chronic synovitis of the knee, with swelling and difficulty of movement.
Calc. Fluor.   A useful remedy in long-standing cases that are slow to respond to treatment.

Teeth

Dentition begins normally at the fourth to sixth month in infancy, and the temporary set of milk teeth, as they are called, should be completed by the thirtieth month. The lower central teeth are the first to erupt followed by the upper central and filling in, in order, towards the back till the set of twenty is complete. During the sixth year the milk teeth begin to shed and the permanent teeth take their place. This set consists of thirty-two teeth and is not complete till the eighteenth to the twentieth year.

Infants frequently have constitutional disturbances during the period of dentition shown by increased irritability or more profound reactions such as diarrhoea, fever or even spasms.

The milk teeth should be cared for as carefully as the permanent ones, as the quality and position of the latter depend on the temporary teeth remaining sound and in place until pushed out by the eruption of the permanent set.

BIOCHEMIC TREATMENT

Calc. Phos.   Teeth develop slowly and decay rapidly. This is the principal nutrition remedy for the teeth. Important for teething infants, children and expectant mothers.

Calc. Fluor.   Enamel of the teeth rough and deficient causing rapid decay, looseness of the teeth in their sockets. Delayed dentition, in alternation with *Calc. Phos.*

Ferr. Phos.   Inflammatory toothache with soreness; bleeding after extractions, in alternation with *Kali. Mur.* when there is swelling.

Kali. Phos.   Bleeding of the gums, severe pain in decayed or filled teeth.

Mag. Phos.   Teeth very sensitive to touch or cold air; severe toothache with shooting pains.

Silica.   Gums painful on slight pressure, gumboils, abscess at the roots.

Calc. Sulph.   Toothache, with inside of gums swollen and sore. Gums bleed on brushing teeth. In alternation with *Silica* for the treatment of gumboils and ulcerations.

See also Combination R.

Tonsillitis

Tonsillitis is an inflammation of the tonsils and may be either acute or chronic. Infection occurs mostly during the winter months. Predisposing factors are similar to those preceding the onset of seasonal coughs and colds. Tonsillitis can be infectious and in children it may be a forerunner of more serious trouble. The onset is sudden with pain in swallowing, chilliness and fever. The tonsils become enlarged and exude a whitish purulent substance and the glands of the throat may become tender and swollen. Medical attention is needed as during the early stages the symptoms are similar to those of diphtheria. There is always a risk of complications in this kind of infection unless proper precautions are taken and this applies particularly with children. The tonsils play an important part in the protective mechanism of the body; they act in the manner of filters and any exudation shows that they are doing their job efficiently.

BIOCHEMIC TREATMENT
Ferr. Phos.   Early stage, fever, flushed face, rapid pulse, vomiting of undigested food.
Kali. Mur.   Second stage, swelling of tonsils, swallowing difficult, tongue white-coated. White or grey spots on tonsils.
Calc. Sulph.   Ulcerating or suppurating tonsillitis, with yellow discharge.
Calc. Phos.   Chronic enlargement of the tonsils, glands swollen and painful. Pain in throat, especially on swallowing.
Silica.   Tonsillitis when the suppurating gland will not heal or, alternatively, to promote suppuration.
Nat. Mur.   Drowsiness, frothy, transparent mucus covering the tonsils. Constant flow of clear saliva; uvula swollen with feeling of obstruction in the throat.
Nat. Phos.   Acid condition of the stomach, creamy yellow mucus on tonsils and base of tongue. Sensation of lump in throat.

Ulcerated Conditions (Mild)
Ulcers are open sores on the surface of the skin or on the surface of any cavity within the body. The process of formation is similar to that of an abscess, since both are inflammatory conditions, but ulceration takes place along a surface. Medical advice should be sought in all cases of ulceration, as the continued presence of any septic condition may lead to more serious trouble.

BIOCHEMIC TREATMENT
Kali. Mur.   Ulceration with a thick, white discharge, bland and not

irritating. Tongue coated white, base of ulcer is usually swollen.
Mouth ulcers.
Silica.   Base of ulcer is spongy, bleeding readily, hard edges,
secretions are thin, yellowish, acrid, pus-like, itching.
Calc. Fluor.   Deep-seated ulceration. Discharge thin, burning.
Varicose ulcers.
Calc. Phos.   Ulcers in persons with weakened constitution; in simple
anaemic conditions.
Calc. Sulph.   Secretions of yellowish pus with blood. Ulcers following
wounds which fail to heal.

Urinary Symptoms

The urinary system comprises the kidneys, which filter the urine
from the blood, two tubes called ureters, through which the urine
flows from the kidneys to the bladder, whence it is avoided through
a further short tube called the urethra. Urine consists chiefly of water
in which are dissolved waste substances resulting from cellular activity.
The amount of water lost daily by the body through perspiration
varies with the season, as is also the case with the kidneys when more
is passed in the winter than in the summer. Regarding the loss of
water by the body, the glands producing perspiration and the kidneys
are complementary to each other. Urine contains about 4 per cent
solids — urea, common salt, phosphates, sulphates, potassium,
sodium, calcium, magnesium, uric acid, ammonia etc. The amount
of urine voided is increased with some diseases and diminished by
others. Similarly the colour of the urine varies according to its chemical
composition — urates cause a reddish-yellow appearance, a greenish
hue is due to the presence of the bile and when blood is present the
colour may be pink or red. Healthy urine will leave a slight deposit
or stain in any vessel in which it has been allowed to stand, due to
the presence of urates, which sometimes become deposited in the
urinary passages in the form of gravel.

Other substances such as albumin may be passed in the urine and
these are discoverable by simple analytical tests. Their detection is
important and early medical advice should be sought whenever
unusual deposits make their appearance. Suppression of the urine
is the state in which the kidneys fail to act and retention describes
the condition when the urine is retained in the bladder. Retention

may be due to obstruction, pressure, nerve weakness, etc., and there should be no delay in calling in the doctor. Prostate gland enlargement can cause blockage of the urethra, a condition common in elderly men (see page 57).

Inability to retain the urine is sometimes due to muscular weakness or nerves and in simple cases the use of the appropriate tissue-salts is helpful, but an examination should always be made first for the presence of any other causative factor.

BIOCHEMIC TREATMENT

Ferr. Phos.   Incontinence of urine, if due to weakness of the sphincter muscle, often seen in women. Irresistible urging to urinate in day-time, aggravated by standing.

Kali. Phos.   Frequent urination and large quantities of urine. Frequently scalding. Incontinence of urine from nervous weakness. Bed wetting in older children.

Mag. Phos.   Constant urgency to urinate when standing or walking. Spasmodic retention of urine.

Calc. Phos.   Bed wetting in young children and old people. Sediment in urine.

Nat. Sulph.   Bed wetting at night or retention of urine. Sandy deposit in urine.

Nat. Mur.   Involuntary urination when walking or coughing. Bed wetting in children with excessive flow of watery urine.

Varicose Veins

Varicose veins are veins that have become stretched and dilated. There are at least two areas in which the veins have a special tendency to become varicose. These are the veins about the lower end of the bowel, producing the condition known as haemorrhoids or piles (see page 48), and the internal saphenous vein, with its branches on the inner side of the leg, knee and thigh. Undoubtedly some people are more liable to the formation of varicose veins than others. A tendency to varicose veins is often hereditary, and jobs that necessitate long-continued standing, with little vigorous muscular exercise can lead to varicose veins. Pregnancy is another common cause of varicose veins, though the condition tends to disappear after the child is born.

BIOCHEMIC TREATMENT

Calc. Fluor. This is the principal remedy when the veins are dilated, also when there is a tendency to varicose ulceration. Bluish discolouration of the tissues.

Ferr. Phos. Inflammation of the veins, red streaks following the course of a vein, throbbing pain along a vein. Alternate with *Calc. Fluor*.

Mag. Phos. Severe acute pains, cramp-like, spasmodic. Alternate with *Calc. Fluor*.

See also 'Elasto'.

Vertigo

Vertigo, or giddiness, may be due to various causes. The ability to balance depends upon sensations derived through the eyes, from touching, but mainly from the semicircular canals of the internal ears. Giddiness may be due to stomach upsets, nausea, headache, etc. Eyesight is a factor and disorders of the circulation may cause a temporary state of bloodlessness of the brain. Getting up suddenly from a sitting or bending position can cause slight giddiness, and elderly people who have to get out of bed during the night should pause momentarily in a sitting position to guard against a sudden faint. Smoking can also be a cause of giddiness. Medical advice should be sought.

BIOCHEMIC TREATMENT

Ferr. Phos. Giddiness from rush of blood to the head, with flushing, throbbing or pressing pain.

Kali. Phos. Giddiness, swimming of the head, from nervous causes, worse when rising or looking upwards.

Nat. Sulph. Giddiness, with bitter taste in the mouth; gastric derangement with inclination to fall on the right side.

Mag. Phos. Vertigo from optical defects, dark spots floating before the eyes.

Nat. Phos. Giddiness with gastric derangements, acidity, loss of appetite. Creamy or golden coating of the tongue. Alternate with *Nat. Sulph.*

Domestic Animals

Many people have been grateful for the benefit that their pets have derived from the biochemic tissue-salts. Their ailments are similar to our own, and their symptoms, viewed biochemically, are a guide to the treatment required. Animals respond well to such corrective measures. They take to this form of medication and their natural mode of living favours a quick response. The common minor ailments of domestic animals can be treated biochemically with most gratifying results but in the event of serious disease, or if the symptoms are in any way unusual, you should immediately consult a veterinary practitioner.

The tissue-salts most frequently needed are:

Ferr. Phos., Kali. Mur. for respiratory disorders; *Kali. Phos.* for highly-strung, nervous animals; *Kali. Sulph.* for skin ailments; *Nat. Mur.* for constipation with dry stools; *Nat. Sulph.* for liverishness, vomiting of bile; *Silica* to improve the condition of the coat and *Calc. Phos.* as a general tonic. The tiny tablets may be given dry on the tongue, or dissolved in a little warm water, or milk. For chronic cases give three daily doses; acute cases, every half hour.

Your Tissue-Salt at a Glance

Remedy	Principal Symptoms
1. Calc. Fluor.	Relaxed conditions, muscular, weakness, poor circulation, dental decay, cracks in the skin.
2. Calc. Phos.	Ill-nourished states, indigestion, chilblains, lowered vitality.
2. Calc. Sulph.	Skin ailments, spots, pimples, wounds that are slow to heal. Has a cleansing action and works well with *Kali. Mur.* and *Nat. Sulph.*
4. Ferr. Phos.	Respiratory ailments, inflammations and congestions, throbbing headaches, feverishness, sore throats, bleeding (apply locally in powder form). An excellent remedy for those conditions associated with advancing years.
5. Kali. Mur.	Congested conditions, thick whitish discharges, respiratory ailments, coughs, colds (alternate with *Ferr. Phos.*).

Note: When you have pin-pointed your tissue-salt, always check your selection by referring to the section headed 'The Twelve Tissue-Salts'.

Remedy	Principal Symptoms
6. Kali. Phos.	Nervous tension, brain-fag, depression, fretfulness, nervous headaches.
7. Kali. Sulph.	Skin ailments, disorders of the scalp, hair, nails and mucous membranes. Catarrh with sticky discharges.
8. Mag. Phos.	Spasmodic, darting pains, cramp, flatulence, neuralgia.
9. Nat. Mur.	Dryness or excessive moisture in any parts of the body, running colds, loss of smell and taste.
10. Nat. Phos.	Acidity, stomach upsets, heartburn, mal-assimilation, rheumatic ailments.
11. Nat. Sulph.	Biliousness, liver upsets, influenza, water retention, rheumatic ailments.
12. Silica.	Pus formation, boils, styes, crippled and brittle nails, scalp disorders.

Note: When you have pin-pointed your tissue-salt, always check your selection by referring to the section headed 'The Twelve Tissue-Salts'.

Prevention is Better than Cure

Without a doubt, prevention is better than cure. Make sure that the means are at hand for dealing with emergencies. By prompt use of the biochemic remedies, early symptoms can often be cleared up. A vast amount of human suffering would be avoided if the right kind of medicinal first aid was on hand at the onset of an illness. As a means of providing this medicinal first aid, the biochemic remedies are ideal. They are pleasant to take and are safe to use at all times. They bring ease by removing the cause of the disease.

'An ounce of prevention is worth a pound of cure.'

Maintenance of Health in Middle Age
Middle age is the period of life when the snap and resilience of former years are no longer in evidence. There may be no serious health problems but there is a tendency to succumb more frequently to minor ailments and these are not so readily shaken off. Consequently, these minor ills must be given attention if they are not to have a cumulative, undermining effect, as a result of seriously disturbed metabolism. Summed up in this phrase, it is probably the real cause of the ageing process.

Metabolism is the conversion of food into living tissue; it is a physiological process of analysis and synthesis. It embraces digestion, assimilation, tissue renovation and the provision of bodily heat and energy, in other words it is the sum total of the biochemic processes.

From this, it becomes obvious that disturbances of metabolism must be avoided and this calls for prompt correction with tissue-salts.

With the onset of middle age, there can follow middle-age spread. This is a clear indication that the entire system needs toning up (*Calc. Fluor.*), digestion and assimilation needs to be improved (*Calc. Phos.*), and excess water to be eliminated from the system (*Nat. Sulph.*). Remember, health cannot be long maintained under excess obesity.

Seasonal Remedies

Spring
Spring is the time of rejuvenation when the body works on a complete cleansing of its own. As a result, it becomes temporarily overcharged with the accumulated impurities thrown off by the tissues. This can give rise to various aches and pains and to that vague out-of-sorts feeling sometimes referred to as 'Spring Fever'. The tissue-salts most helpful at this season of the year to assist Nature's spring-cleaning are *Calc. Phos.* to tone up the system and bring renewed vigour and vitality to the newly-cleansed tissues. Next, *Ferr. Phos.* to increase the properties of the blood and so enable it more quickly to dispose of trouble making waste matter. And *Nat. Phos.* the acid neutraliser, which has a soothing effect throughout the whole alimentary tract, helping to improve digestion and assimilation.

Avoiding Summer Ills
The carefree days of summer can so easily be overclouded by digestive and gastric upsets. These ailments are most common in summertime and may be caused by sudden changes of diet, unaccustomed foods, chills in the stomach following bodily overheating, exposure to hot sunshine etc.

   Kali. Mur., *Nat. Phos.* and *Nat. Sulph.* help to safeguard summer health. All are excellent digestive aids. *Kali. Mur.* is the tissue-salt concerned with the production of saliva, a secretion of great importance in the early stages of digestion. It also offsets the possible ill-effects of rich fatty foods. Lack of appetite calls for *Kali. Mur. Nat. Phos.* is the acid neutraliser. *Nat. Sulph.* largely controls the healthy functioning of the liver. It ensures an adequate supply of free-flowing healthy bile, so necessary for the later stages of digestion. *See also Combination S.*

Autumn and Winter
During the autumn and winter months, sudden changes of temperature, chilly damp nights, harsh inclement weather produce

coughs, colds, sore throats and other respiratory ailments. Resistance to such ailments can be improved by taking *Ferr. Phos.*, *Kali. Mur.*, and *Nat. Mur.*

Ferr. Phos. is needed for the feverishness, stuffiness and sneezing that herald the onset of a cold. This tissue-salt corrects inflammatory tendencies and prevents local congestion. *Kali. Mur.* has to do with congestions and catarrh. It helps to bring about the elimination of harmful waste matter which, if allowed to remain clogging the tissues, would render those tissues liable to infection.

Nat. Mur. also plays an important part in the elimination of the waste products of cellular activity. It controls the degree of moisture in the tissues. The need for *Nat. Mur.* is readily recognized in what is known as a 'running cold'. *See also Combination Q.*

Your Questions Answered

Q. I have so many symptoms that I am puzzled to know which remedy to try first. Supposing I choose the wrong remedy?

A. Ask yourself which is the predominant symptom and concentrate on that in the first instance. If, for example, it is a throbbing recurrent headache, or a pain with inflammation, the best choice would be *Ferr. Phos.* No harm, however, would follow if the wrong remedy were selected, as the body will simply excrete what it does not require for balanced cell nutrition.

Q. I have heard so much about the tissue-salts from my friends who tell me how good these remedies can be. But I hesitate to try them myself because I am taking other medication. Is there any risk of the tissue-salts conflicting?

A. The answer to this is you can always, with perfect safety, take the tissue-salts in conjunction with other medicines. In fact, the tissue-salts can often be used with advantage to supplement other treatment.

Q. I am what is politely termed 'a senior citizen'. Am I too old to benefit from the biochemic tissue-salts?

A. No! Young and old alike respond to the tissue-salts, though with advancing years, the body's recuperative powers tend to slow down. There is no need, however, to wait for a full recovery to enjoy a measure of relief.

Q. I'm a bad traveller. Can any of the tissue-salts help me?

A. Yes! Take *Nat. Phos.* and *Kali. Phos.*, two doses of each, before starting the journey; whilst travelling at half-hourly intervals as a preventative.

Q. I have taken several biochemic remedies and they all look and taste alike. Why is that?

A. This is because the bulk of the tablets is composed of lactose (sugar of milk) which is purely an inert base.

Q. Is there any relationship between the tissue-salts and herbal remedies?

A. They are different branches of medicine, but they work well together, as both are based upon the application of Nature's laws of health and healing. In fact, the tissue-salts are present in some herbal remedies.

Q. I wish to consult a homoeopathic doctor. How do I go about this?

A. You can obtain the name and address of your nearest homoeopathic doctor by writing to the Secretary, British Homoeopathic Association, 27a Devonshire Street, London, W1 (Tel No 01-935-2163).

Q. Do the Biochemic Remedies keep indefinitely?

A. Yes! provided they are properly stored. They should be kept in a dry place away from strong smelling substances such as camphor, vapour rubs etc. The caps should always be firmly replaced after use.

Q. I suffer from intermittent headaches. Should I take the biochemic treatment continuously or only when the headaches occur?

A. The answer to this is that the biochemic remedies should be taken continuously until the symptoms undergoing treatment have cleared up. They are not suppressants and are cumulative in their action.

Note: *This programme particularly applies to conditions such as menstrual pain, hay fever, piles, neuralgia etc.*

Q. The tissue-salts have a sweetish taste. My wife is a diabetic can she take these remedies with perfect sfaety?

A. Yes! Although the tissue-salts are triturated in a base of lactose (sugar of milk) the sugar content of the tablets is so very tiny that no reaction should be experienced.

✗ Not really

Combination Remedies

Combined formulations of the tissue-salts were unknown in Schuessler's day. Over the years, however, the convenience and effectiveness of the combined formulations of the tissue-salts has come to be recognized. They do make remedy selection easier, and there is no doubt at all that, in general, combined remedies are as effective as single tissue-salts.

The foremost manufacturer and distributor of the Schuessler tissue-salts in the U.K., New Era Laboratories, 39 Wales Farm Road, London W3 6XH, supply a comprehensive range of combination remedies (see below). These remedies have been specially formulated for use in certain groups of ailments, and are the result of many years of clinical experience.

A. *Ferr. Phos., Kali. Phos., Mag. Phos.*
   For sciatica, neuralgia and neuritis.
   The sciatic nerve runs from the lower back, through the buttock and down the back of the entire leg. Sciatica is pain along the whole or part of the course of this nerve. Combination A can be usefully taken in addition to any other methods that might have to be employed to relieve the pain.

B. *Calc. Phos., Kali. Phos., Ferr. Phos.*
   For general debility, nervous exhaustion.
   Sometimes life can make us feel nervy and generally rather 'drained'. This feeling is quite common too during convalescence from any ailment, operation or injury. Combination B can help smooth over these feelings.

C. *Mag. Phos.*, *Nat. Phos.*, *Nat. Sulph.*, *Silica.*
   For acidity, heartburn and dyspepsia.

   Sufferers from indigestion or dyspepsia will know all about the consequent uncomfortable symptoms. One of these is acidity caused by over-production of stomach acid. Another is heartburn, a scalding or burning sensation behind the breastbone, usually caused by regurgitation of stomach acid. Combination C is designed to help with these symptoms either individually or combined.

D. *Kali. Mur.*, *Kali. Sulph.*, *Calc. Sulph.*, *Silica.*
   For minor skin ailments.

   Skin ailments which are too minor to concern your doctor can still be troublesome and annoying to you. When you want a natural remedy for such skin troubles Combination D could be helpful. It is best taken as a course of treatment.

E. *Calc. Phos.*, *Mag. Phos.*, *Nat. Phos.*, *Nat. Sulph.*
   For flatulence, colic and indigestion.

   Flatulence is a highly unpleasant distension of the stomach or intestines with air or gases. It can itself lead to colicky pains, though these are often the result of indigestion. Whether these or other symptoms of indigestion occur singly or together they can be eased by the particular combination of tissue-salts present in Combination E.

F. *Kali. Phos.*, *Mag. Phos.*, Nat. Mur., *Silica.*
   For nervous headaches and migraine.

   Nervous headaches are usually brought on by an upset and can be so disabling. Migraine headaches are periodic throbbing headaches which usually start on one side. They are brought on by a variety of causes, often certain foods. The trigger differs from person to person. With the migraine headache it is wise to see the doctor to make sure there is no organic cause. Sufferers from nervous and migraine headaches can frequently be helped by Combination F.

G. *Calc. Fluor., Calc. Phos., Kali. Phos., Nat. Mur.*
   For backache, lumbago and piles.

   At some time in their life most people experience backache.
   Lumbago is backache in the lumbar region of the spine. Backache
   seems to dominate life when present and so sufferers may be glad
   to try Combination G.

H. *Mah. Phos., Nat. Mur., Silica.*
   For hay fever and allergic rhinitis

   Hay fever is an 'allergic' condition of the mucous membranes
   of the nose, eyes and upper respiratory tract. It is common in
   both sexes and in all age groups, but is very treatable by
   Combination H, particularly if treatment is started from six
   weeks before the expected onset of normal symptoms.

I. *Ferr. Phos., Kali. Sulph., Mag. Phos.*
   For fibrositis and muscular pain.

   Fibrositis and muscular pain (sometimes called muscular
   rheumatism) is marked by pain and stiffness. It is caused by
   inflammation of the sheaths surrounding the muscle fibres which
   are involved with body movement. Combination I provides three
   biochemic tissue-salts which act together favourably for this
   condition. Naturally if the trouble persists medical help should
   be sought.

J. *Ferr. Phos., Kali. Mur., Nat. Mur.*
   For coughs, colds and chestiness.

   The common cold with its unpleasant symptoms of running
   or stuffy nose, sneezing and catarrh is often 'caught' when the
   body's resistance is lowered by exposure to cold or wet. Often
   these symptoms are followed by a cough and slight chestiness.
   Should bronchitis develop or the cough persist the advice of a
   doctor should be sought. The symptoms of a common cold can
   be eased by Combination J.

K. *Kali. Sulph., Nat. Mur., Silica.*
   Brittle nails and falling hair.

   Hair grows from follicles in the skin which are nourished by
   blood vessels. The appearance and health of the hair often reflects

the health of the body as a whole. Nails grow from the nail beds on fingers and toes and they have a protective function. During illness nails may cease to grow and Combination K has a particular combination of three tissue-salts which are relevant to different aspects of the maintenance of hair and nail health.

L. *Calc. Fluor., Ferr. Phos., Nat. Mur.*
For varicose veins and circulatory disorders.

The three tissue-salts in Combination L act synergistically, which means that each reinforces the action of the other. Taken regularly they may help maintain some aspects of the health of those leading a sedentary lifestyle.

M. *Calc. Phos., Kali. Mur., Nat. Phos., Nat. Sulph.*
For rheumatism.

Almost everyone in the U.K. experiences rheumatic pain at some time in his or her life. If persistent or severe, medical help should be sought, but in many instances self-help with a safe home treatment will be adequate. Combination M is just such a suitable home treatment.

N. *Calc. Phos., Kali. Mur., Kali. Phos., Mag. Phos.*
For menstrual pain.

Menstrual pain (dysmenorrhoea) refers to the pain experienced during the monthly period. It can vary in intensity from month to month, and may occur at different times during the blood flow. Always seek medical advice if pain is severe or there is doubt or anxiety about a possible organic cause for the pain, or there is excessive blood flow or clotting. Combination N causes no side-effects and so can be taken with confidence by menstruating women of all ages.

P. *Calc. Fluor., Calc. Phos., Kali. Phos., Mag. Phos.*
For aching feet and legs.

For those who spend much of the day standing, particularly standing still, aching feet and tired legs are a common phenomenon. Combination P is a particularly appropriate remedy for such problems, although it should be borne in mind that the troubles can often arise from wearing unsuitable shoes.

Q. *Ferr. Phos., Kali. Mur., Kali. Sulph., Nat. Mur.*
   For catarrh and sinus disorders.
   Catarrh is the troublesome discharge formed as a result of inflammation of the mucous membranes at the back of the nose. Often it is associated with a concomitant upset in the sinuses. Combination Q incorporates four biochemic tissue-salts to help relieve these symptoms.

R. *Calc. Fluor., Calc. Phos., Ferr. Phos., Mag. Phos., Silica.*
   For infants' teething pains.
   Many infants experience some difficulty with teething. As the erupting tooth forces its way through the tender gum it can cause pain and stress to the baby. Combination R has been designed to help alleviate these infant teething pains.

S. *Kali. Mur., Nat. Phos., Nat. Sulph.*
   For sick headaches, stomach upsets and biliousness.
   Stomach upsets are often accompanied by biliousness and sick headaches. Though usually lasting only a day or two, these upsets can be most unpleasant. Combination S can be used when the above troubles occur together or when each occurs alone.

'New Era' Proprietary Biochemic Remedies
These are:
Elasto, Nervone and Zief.

Elasto	*Calc. Fluor., Calc. Phos., Ferr. Phos., Mag. Phos.*	
	For varicose veins, aching legs and allied conditions.	
Nervone	*Calc. Phos., Kali. Mur., Kali. Phos., Mag. Phos., Nat. Phos.*	
	For nervous debility, nerve pains and allied conditions.	
Zief	*Ferr. Phos., Nat. Phos., Nat. Sulph., Silica.*	
	For rheumatic pain and allied conditions.	

Elasto derives its name from elastin which is the material used in the repair and maintenance of all the elastic tissues of the body, notably the blood vessels. Elasto promotes the formation of elastin and thus acts as a powerful aid in overcoming relaxed conditions whenever they occur. When the elastic quality of the blood vessels is unimpaired, circulation is free and efficient; the blood is enriched and an adequate supply of life-giving oxygen reaches the tissues. Elasto was first marketed in the late 1920's. It was unique — an effective internal treatment for varicose veins. Elasto soon became a household word. One of its advertising slogans was 'Whatever your walk in life, Elasto will stop you limping.' Reports from users of this product support that statement. So if you suffer from leg troubles, take Elasto and stop limping.

Nervone was a later arrival and quickly established a reputation as being a safe and reliable remedy for nerve troubles, neuralgic pain, want of energy etc. Two of its active constituents are *Kali. Phos.* and *Mag. Phos. Calc. Phos.* is included in the formulation for its tonic effective and restorative properties; also *Kali. Mur.* Finally, *Nat. Phos.*, the acid neutraliser is added for its soothing influence on the gastric system.

Zief was first welcomed by rheumatic sufferers in 1964. It is a combination of four tissue-salts which are indicated for the treatment of rheumatic conditions. Zief has proved effective in giving progressive relief from rheumatic pain and, dare it be said, arthritic sufferers have reported that they have derived benefit from this remedy. On the other hand, to be equally truthful, some arthritic sufferers have not found Zief helpful, which is not surprising for arthritis is a tough proposition.

Repertory of Symptoms and their Corresponding Remedies

HEAD

Dandruff: *Nat. Mur.*, *Kali. Sulph.*
Hair, falling out of: *Kali. Sulph.*, *Silica*, *Nat. Mur.*
Headache accompanied by:
  biliousness, bitter taste: *Nat. Sulph.*
  constipation: *Nat. Mur.*, *Kali. Mur.*
  drowsiness: *Nat. Mur.*
  dull, heavy hammering: *Nat. Mur.*, *Ferr. Phos.*
  irritability: *Kali. Phos.*
  pain in temples: *Ferr. Phos.*, *Nat. Phos.*
    over eye: *Ferr. Phos.*
    throbbing, beating: *Ferr. Phos.*
  profusion of tears: *Nat. Mur.*
  sharp, shooting pains: *Mag. Phos.*
  tearful mood: *Kali. Phos.*
  thick white coating on the tongue: *Kali. Mur.*
  unrefreshing sleep: *Nat. Mur.*
  vomiting of acid sour fluids: *Nat. Phos.*
  vomiting of frothy phlegm: *Nat. Mur.*
  vomiting of undigested food: *Ferr. Phos.*
Headache:
  from mental work: *Kali. Phos.*
  in nervous subjects: *Kali. Phos.*
  neuralgic: *Kali. Phos.*, *Mag. Phos.*
  on awakening in the morning: *Nat. Phos.*
    crown of head: *Nat. Phos.*
  rheumatic, evening aggravation: *Kali. Sulph.*
Headache relieved by:

cheerful excitement: *Kali. Phos.*
cool air: *Kali. Sulph.*
Migraine: *Kali. Phos.*, *Mag. Phos.*, *Nat. Sulph.*
Neuralgia of head, when pain is sharp: *Mag. Phos.*
Neuralgic headache, with humming in the ears: *Kali. Phos.*
Sick headache, arising from sluggish action of the liver: *Kali. Mur.*
  with vomiting of undigested food: *Ferr. Phos.*
  with bitter taste in the mouth, vomiting of bile: *Nat. Sulph.*
    vomiting of sour fluids: *Nat. Phos.*
Trembling and involuntary shaking of the head: *Mag. Phos.*
Vertigo from excessive secretions of bile, tongue has a dirty greenish
    or greenish-brown coating at the back part, bitter taste in the
    mouth: *Nat. Sulph.*
  from exhaustion and weakness: *Kali. Phos.*

MENTAL STATES

Children, crying and screaming: *Kali. Phos.*
  ill-tempered: *Kali. Phos.*
Depressed spirits: *Kali. Phos.*, *Calc. Phos.*, *Nat. Mur.*
Desire for solitude: *Calc. Phos.*, *Kali. Phos.*
Fainting of nervous persons: *Kali. Phos.*
  tendency to: *Kali. Phos.*
Fits of crying: *Kali. Phos.*
  laughing: *Kali. Phos.*
Hopeless, with dejected spirits: *Nat. Mur.*
Impatience and nervousness: *Kali. Phos.*
Irritability: *Kali. Phos.*
Memory, poor: *Calc. Phos.*, *Kali. Phos.*, *Mag. Phos.*
Moods, anxious: *Kali. Phos.*
Moods, gloomy: *Kali. Phos.*
Sensitiveness: *Kali. Phos.*
Shyness: *Kali. Phos.*
Sleepiness: *Nat. Mur.*
Weeps easily: *Nat. Mur.*

EYES

Dimness of sight from weakness of the optic nerve: *Kali. Phos.*

Discharge, golden-yellow, creamy: *Nat. Phos.*
   thick white mucus: *Kali. Mur.*
   yellow: *Calc. Sulph.*
   greenish, serous: *Kali. Sulph.*
   slimy secretions: *Kali. Sulph.*
Drooping of lids: *Kali. Phos.*, *Mag. Phos.*
Eyes, bloodshot: *Ferr. Phos.*
   glued together in the morning, with a creamy discharge: *Nat. Phos.*
Flow of tears from the eyes when associated with colds in the head:
     Nat. Mur.
   with neuralgic pains in the eye: *Nat. Mur.*, *Mag. Phos.*
Granulations on eyelids: *Ferr. Phos.*, *Kali. Mur.*, *Nat. Mur.*
Neuralgic pain in the eyes, with flow of tears: *Nat. Mur.*
Smarting secretions, with tears: *Nat. Mur.*
Sore eyes, with specks of white matter on the lids: *Kali. Mur.*
Spasmodic twitching of lids: *Mag. Phos.*
Stoppage of tear ducts from the cold: *Nat. Mur.*
Stye on lids: *Silica.*
Weak eyes, with tears when going into the cold air: *Nat. Mur.*

EARS

Catarrh of ear, causing deafness: *Kali. Sulph.*, *Kali. Mur.*
   involving Eustachian tubes: *Kali. Sulph.*, *Kali. Mur.*
     middle ear: *Ferr. Phos.*, *Kali. Mur.*
Cracking noises in ear on blowing nose: *Kali. Mur.*
   when swallowing: *Kali. Mur.*
Difficulty of hearing, accompanied by exhaustion of nervous system:
     Kali. Phos.
   from swelling of Eustachian tubes: *Kali. Mur.*, *Kali. Sulph.*
Earache, accompanied by:
   beating, throbbing pain: *Ferr. Phos.*
   swelling of Eustachian tube; glands or tonsils: *Kali. Mur.*
   yellow, mattery discharge: *Kali. Sulph.*
Exudations from ear, thick, white and moist: *Kali. Mur.*
Glands around the ear swollen; noises in the ear; snapping and
     cracking: *Kali. Mur.*
Heat and burning of the ears, with gastric symptoms: *Nat. Phos.*

Inflammation of the ears, first stage for the fever and pain: *Ferr. Phos.*

NOSE

Bleeding from the nose: *Ferr. Phos.*
  blackish or coagulating: *Kali. Phos.*
Catarrh, accompanied by fever: *Ferr. Phos.*
  aggravated in evening: *Kali. Sulph.*
  dry, with stuffy sensation: *Kali. Mur.*
Discharge, albuminous: *Calc. Phos.*
  clear, watery, transparent mucus: *Nat. Mur.*
  lumpy, yellow, tough: *Calc. Fluor.*
  purulent, bloody: *Calc. Sulph.*
  slimy, yellow, watery, greenish: *Kali. Sulph.*
  thick and white: *Kali. Mur.*
  yellow, creamy: *Nat. Phos.*
  yellow, offensive: *Nat. Phos.*
Dryness of nose, with scabbing: *Nat. Mur.*, *Silica.*
Edges of nostrils itch: *Silica.*
First or inflammatory stage of colds: *Ferr. Phos.*
Frequent sneezing: *Silica.*, *Nat. Mur.*
Hawking and spitting, constant: *Calc. Phos.*
Hay Fever: *Nat. Mur.*, *Mag. Phos.*
Loss of smell or perversion of the sense of smell, not connected with
    a cold: *Mag. Phos.*
  with dryness and rawness of the pharynx: *Nat. Mur.*
Nose, inflamed at edges of nostrils: *Silica.*
Pharynx, dryness and rawness of: *Nat. Mur.*
Polypi: *Calc. Phos.*
Sneezing: *Nat. Mur.*
Stuffy cold in head, with yellow, lumpy mucus: *Calc. Fluor.*
  with collection of greenish mucus: *Kali. Sulph.*, *Silica.*

FACE

Acne: *Calc. Sulph.*
Beard, tender pimples under: *Calc. Sulph.*
Chaps of lips: *Calc. Fluor.*
Face flushed, cold sensation at nape of neck: *Ferr. Phos.*

Feeling of coldness or numbness of face: *Calc. Phos.*
Feverish complexion: *Ferr. Phos.*
Inflammatory neuralgia of the face: *Ferr. Phos.*
Lightning-like pains in face: *Mag. Phos.*
Neuralgia, accompanied by:
    flow of tears: *Nat. Mur.*
    shifting pains: Kali. Sulph.
    shooting pains: *Mag. Phos.*
    spasmodic pains: *Mag. Phos.*
Neuralgia:
    aggravated by cold: *Mag. Phos.*
    with exhaustion of nervous system: *Kali. Phos.*
    relieved by hot applications: *Mag. Phos.*
Nodules on face: *Calc. Sulph.*
Pale face in children when teething is difficult: *Calc. Phos.*
Pimples on face, mattery: *Calc. Sulph.*
    at age of puberty: *Calc. Sulph., Calc. Phos.*
Yellow, sallow, or jaundiced face due to biliousness: *Nat. Sulph.*

THROAT

Choking on attempting to swallow: *Mag. Phos.*
Constricted feeling of throat: *Mag. Phos.*
Constant hoarseness: *Calc. Phos.*
Dry red and inflamed throat: *Ferr. Phos.*
First stage of sore throat, when there is pain, heat and redness: *Ferr. Phos.*
Glands, painful, aching: *Calc. Phos.*
Hoarseness, constant: *Calc. Phos., Ferr. Phos.*
Inflammation, of the mucous lining of the throat, with watery secretions: *Nat. Mur.*
    of tonsils: *Ferr. Phos.*
        with greyish-white patches: *Kali. Mur.*
Larynx, burning and soreness in: *Calc. Phos., Ferr. Phos.*
    closing of, by spasm: *Mag. Phos.*
    lump in, on swallowing: *Nat. Sulph.*
Loss of voice, from strain: *Ferr. Phos.*
Pharynx, burning and soreness in: *Calc. Phos.*
Raw feeling in throat: *Nat. Phos.*

Redness and inflammation: *Ferr. Phos.*
Relaxed condition of: *Calc. Fluor.*
Sore throat, as if a plug had lodged in the throat: *Nat. Mur.*
  of singers and speakers: *Ferr. Phos.*
  with excessive dryness or too much secretion: *Nat. Mur.*
Stinging sore throat, only when swallowing, the neck being painful
     to touch: *Silica.*
Suppuration of throat: *Calc. Sulph.*
Swallowing, painful: *Ferr. Phos.*
Tonsillitis, after pus has begun to form: *Silica.*
Tonsils, chronic enlargement of: *Calc. Phos.*
  creamy, yellow, moist coating on: *Nat. Phos.*
  grey-white patches on: *Kali. Mur.*
  inflamed: *Ferr. Phos.*
Ulcerations, with thick yellow discharges: *Silica.*
Ulcerated throat, white or grey patches: *Kali. Mur.*
Windpipe, spasmodic closing: *Mag. Phos.*

MOUTH

Acid taste in mouth: *Nat. Phos.*
Bad taste in mouth: *Nat. Sulph., Kali. Phos.*
  in morning: *Calc. Phos.*
Bitter taste in mouth: *Nat. Sulph.*
Constant hawking of slimy mucus: *Nat. Sulph.*
  spitting of frothy mucus: *Nat. Mur.*
Cracked lips: *Calc. Fluor.*
Creamy, yellow coating at back part of roof of mouth: *Nat. Phos.*
Glands and gums swollen: *Kali. Mur.*
Gums hot, swollen, and inflamed: *Ferr. Phos.*
Hard swelling on jaw-bones: *Calc. Fluor.*
Hawking, constant, of foul, slimy mucus from trachea and stomach:
     Nat. Sulph.
Inflammation of salivary glands, when secreting excessive amount
     of saliva: *Nat. Mur.*
Mouth full of thick, greenish-white, tenacious slime: *Nat. Sulph.*
Rawness of mouth: *Kali. Mur.*
Saliva, excess of: *Nat. Mur.*

Sour taste in mouth: *Nat. Phos.*
Thrush, in children: *Kali. Mur.*
  with much saliva: *Nat. Mur.*
Twitching, spasmodic, of lips: *Mag. Phos.*
Ulcers in mouth, ash-grey: *Kali. Phos.*
  corners of mouth: *Silica.*
  white: *Kali. Mur.*
Very offensive breath: *Kali. Phos.*

TONGUE

Blisters on tip of tongue: *Nat. Mur.*, *Calc. Phos.*
Chronic swelling of tongue: *Calc. Fluor.*
Coating on tongue, clear slimy, watery: *Nat. Mur.*
  dirty, greenish-grey, bitter taste: *Nat. Sulph.*
  golden-yellw, on back part: *Nat. Phos.*
  greyish-white: *Kali. Mur.*
  like stale brownish, liquid mustard: *Kali. Phos.*
  moist, creamy on back part: *Nat. Phos.*
  yellow and slimy: *Kali. Sulph.*
Cracked appearance of tongue: *Calc. Fluor.*
Dark red and inflamed tongue: *Ferr. Phos.*
Frothy bubbles on edges of tongue: *Nat. Mur.*
Induration of tongue, after inflammation: *Silica*, *Calc. Fluor.*
Inflammation of tongue: *Ferr. Phos.*, *Kali. Mur.*
Numbness of tongue: *Calc. Phos.*
Pimples on tip of tongue: *Calc. Phos.*
Swollen tongue: *Kali. Mur.*, *Calc. Phos.*
Ulcers on tongue: *Silica.*
Vesicles on tongue: *Nat. Mur.*

TEETH AND GUMS

Decay of teeth as soon as they appear: *Calc. Phos.*
Dentition, retarded: *Calc. Phos.*
Enamel, brittle: *Calc. Fluor.*
  rough and thin: *Calc. Fluor.*
Gastric derangements during teething: *Nat. Phos.*
Gums, bleed easily: *Kali. Phos.*
  pale: *Calc. Phos.*

Gumboil: *Silica.*
  before pus begins to form: *Kali. Mur.*
Infants, teething of, with drooling: *Nat. Mur.*
Rapid decay of teeth: *Calc. Fluor., Calc. Phos.*
Teeth, sensitive to cold air: *Mag. Phos.*
  loose in sockets: *Calc. Fluor.*
  to touch: *Mag. Phos., Calc. Fluor.*
Toothache accompanied by:
  excessive flow of saliva or of tears: *Nat. Mur.*
  neuralgia of face: *Mag. Phos.*
  swelling of gums or cheeks: *Kali. Mur., Ferr. Phos.*
  ulceration: *Silica.*
Toothache:
  aggravated by hot liquids: *Ferr. Phos.*
  relieved by cold applications: *Ferr. Phos.*
    hot applications: *Mag. Phos.*
Ulceration of roots of teeth: *Calc. Sulph.*

GASTRIC SYMPTOMS

Abnormal appetite, but food causes distress: *Calc. Phos.*
Acid drinks aggravate the stomach: *Mag. Phos.*
Belching, brings back taste of food: *Ferr. Phos.*
  sour eructation: *Nat. Phos.*
Biliousness from too much bile: *Nat. Sulph.*
Bloated, stomach feels: *Calc. Phos.*
Catarrh of the stomach, with yellow, slimy tongue: *Kali. Sulph.*
Cold drinks relieve symptoms: *Ferr. Phos.*
  aggravate symptoms: *Calc. Phos., Mag. Phos.*
Craving for salt or salty food: *Nat. Mur.*
Excess of salvia; tongue has a clear, frothy, transparent coating: *Nat. Mur.*
Fatty food disagrees with the digestive system: *Kali. Mur., Nat. Phos.*
Flatulence, with distress about heart: *Kali. Phos., Nat. Phos.*
  with sluggishness of the liver: *Kali. Mur., Nat. Sulph.*
Heartburn: *Calc. Phos., Nat. Sulph., Silica.*
Hiccups: *Mag. Phos.*

Indigestion, accompanied by griping pains: *Mag. Phos.*
  vomiting of greasy, white, opaque mucus: *Kali. Mur.*
  watery vomiting and salty taste in the mouth: *Nat. Mur.*
  with pain in the stomach and watery gathering in the mouth, or sour
      taste in the mouth: *Nat. Mur.*
  with pressure and fullness at the pit of the stomach: *Kali. Sulph.*
Lumpiness, food lies in a lump: *Calc. Phos.*
Morning sickness: *Nat. Mur.*, *Nat. Phos.*, *Nat. Sulph.*
Nausea, with sour risings: *Nat. Phos.*
  'gone' sensation in the stomach: *Kali. Phos.*
Salty taste in mouth: *Nat. Mur.*
Travel sickness: *Kali. Phos.*, *Nat. Phos.*
Sick headache from gastric derangements: *Nat. Sulph.*
Sour, acid risings: *Nat. Phos.*
Vomiting, after cold drinks: *Calc. Phos.*
  bile: *Nat. Sulph.*
  sour acid fluids: *Nat. Phos.*
  thick white phlegm: *Kali. Mur.*
  undigested food: *Ferr. Phos.*
Waterbrash: *Nat. Mur.*

ABDOMEN

Abdomen, bloated: *Kali. Sulph.*, *Mag. Phos.*
  distended: *Mag. Phos.*, *Nat. Sulph.*
Anus, itching at: *Nat. Phos.*, *Calc. Fluor.*
  cracks and fissures of the: *Calc. Fluor.*
Colic of infants: *Mag. Phos.*
Constant urging to stool: *Kali. Mur.*
Constipation, see stools.
Diarrhoea, see stools.
Faeces, inability to expel: *Calc. Fluor.*
Flatulence, with pains in left side: *Kali. Phos.*
Flatulent colic: *Nat. Phos.*, *Nat. Sulph.*, *Mag. Phos.*
Liver, sluggish: *Kali. Mur.*
Sulphurous odour of gas from bowels: *Kali. Sulph.*

STOOLS

Constipation, from dryness of the mucous membrane: *Nat. Mur.*
  light-coloured stool, showing want of bile; sluggish action of the
      liver: *Kali. Mur.*
Diarrhoea, after eating greasy, fatty food: *Kali. Mur.*
  alternating with constipation: *Nat. Mur.*
  especially of children, with green, sour-smelling stools caused by
      an acid condition: *Nat. Phos.*
  in teething children; stools slimy, green, undigested: *Calc. Phos.*
  like water: *Nat. Mur.*
  with greenish, bilious stools or vomiting of bile: *Nat. Sulph.*
  with pale, yellow, clay-coloured stool, swelling of the abdomen,
      slimy stools: *Kali. Mur.*
  putrid, foul evacuations, depression and exhaustion of the nerves:
      Kali. Phos.
  yellow, slimy, purulent matter: *Kali. Sulph.*
Flatulent colic, with green, sour-smelling stools: *Nat. Phos.*
Frequent call for stool, but passes nothing: *Calc. Phos.*
Loose morning stool, worse in cold wet weather: *Nat. Sulph.*
Looseness of bowels, in old people: *Nat. Sulph.*
  with watery stools: *Nat. Mur.*
Retention of stool: *Nat. Mur.*
Stool is hot, often noisy and offensive: *Calc. Phos.*
Stools are dry and often produce fissures in the rectum: *Nat. Mur.*

FEMALE ORGANS
(See Female Disorders
Pages 40-45)

URINARY SYMPTOMS

Cystitis: *Kali. Mur.*, *Ferr. Phos.*, *Kali. Phos.*, *Mag. Phos.*
Enuresis of children (wetting of the bed): *Kali. Phos.*, *Nat. Phos.*,
      Ferr. Phos., *Nat. Mur.*, *Calc. Phos.*
Excessive flow of watery urine: *Nat. Mur.*
Frequent passing of much water, sometimes scalding: *Kali. Phos.*
Great thirst, with excessive flow of watery urine: *Nat. Mur.*
Inability to retain urine, from nervous debility: *Kali. Phos.*

Incontinence, weakness of sphincter: *Ferr. Phos.*
Involuntary emission of urine while walking or coughing: *Nat. Mur.*
Sandy deposits in urine: *Nat. Sulph.*
Spasmodic retention of urine: *Mag. Phos.*

RESPIRATORY ORGANS

Acute, painful, short, irritating cough: *Ferr. Phos.*
All inflammatory conditions of the respiratory tract, in the first stage: *Ferr. Phos.*
Asthma, accompanied by laboured breathing: *Kali. Phos.*, *Mag. Phos.*
Asthma, aggravated by damp weather: *Nat. Sulph.*
  bronchial: *Kali. Sulph.*, *Calc. Phos.*
Children, cough of teething: *Calc. Phos.*
Cold in chest: *Ferr. Phos.*
Constant spitting of frothy water: *Nat. Mur.*
Convulsive fits of coughing: *Mag. Phos.*
Cough, better in cool open air: *Kali. Sulph.*
Cough, hard, dry: *Ferr. Phos.*
  irritating, painful: *Ferr. Phos.*
  worse in evening: *Kali. Sulph.*
    warm room: *Kali. Sulph.*
Croupy hoarseness: *Kali. Mur.*, *Kali. Sulph.*
Expectoration, albuminous: *Calc. Phos.*
  salty: *Nat. Mur.*
  slips back: *Kali. Sulph.*
  thick, yellow, green: *Silica.*
  tiny, yellow lumps: *Calc. Fluor.*
  watery: *Nat. Mur.*
  yellow, green, slimy: *Kali. Sulph.*
Hay fever: *Mag. Phos.*, *Nat. Mur.*, *Silica.*
Hawking, to clear throat: *Calc. Phos.*
Hoarseness, from cold: *Kali. Mur.*, *Ferr. Phos.*
  of speakers: *Ferr. Phos.*
  over-exertion of voice: *Ferr. Phos.*
Loud noisy cough: *Kali. Mur.*
Rattling in chest: *Kali. Mur.*, *Nat. Mur.*
Shortness of breath from asthma or with exhaustion or want of proper nerve power: *Kali. Phos.*, *Mag. Phos.*

Soreness of chest: *Ferr. Phos.*
Spasmodic cough: *Mag. Phos.*
  worse lying down: *Mag. Phos.*
Stomach cough, thick, tenacious, white phlegm: *Kali. Mur.*
Tickling in throat: *Calc. Fluor.*

CIRCULATORY SYMPTOMS

Anaemia: *Ferr. Phos., Calc. Phos.*
Blood, thin, watery: *Nat. Mur.*
  thick, clotting: *Kali. Mur.*
Circulation, poor: *Kali. Phos., Calc. Phos., Calc. Fluor.*

BACK AND EXTREMITIES

Chilblains on hands and feet: *Calc. Phos., Kali. Phos., Kali. Mur.*
Cracking of joints: *Nat. Phos.*
Gout: *Nat. Phos., Nat. Sulph., Ferr. Phos.*
Lumbago: *Calc. Phos., Ferr. Phos., Nat. Phos.*
  from strains: *Calc. Fluor.*
Nails, brittle: *Silica, Kali. Sulph., Calc. Fluor.*
Neck, muscles stiff: *Ferr. Phos.*
Rheumatism: *Ferr. Phos., Nat. Phos., Nat. Sulph., Silica.*
  with swelling: *Kali. Mur.*
Sciatica: *Mag. Phos., Ferr. Phos.*
Sprains: *Ferr. Phos.*
Strains: *Ferr. Phos.*
Trembling and involuntary motion of the hands: *Mag. Phos.*
Varicose veins and ulcerations: *Calc. Fluor.*

NERVOUS SYMPTOMS

Cries easily: *Kali. Phos.*
Despondent: *Kali. Phos.*
Dwells upon grievances: *Kali. Phos.*
Feet twitch during sleep: *Nat. Sulph.*
Hands twitch during sleep: *Nat. Sulph.*
Head, involuntary shaking of: *Mag. Phos.*
Involuntary motion of hands: *Mag. Phos.*

Neuralgia accompanied by:
  congestion, after taking cold: *Ferr. Phos.*
  depression: *Kali. Phos.*
  failure of strength: *Kali. Phos.*
  flow of saliva: *Nat. Mur.*
  flow of tears: *Nat. Mur.*
  shifting pains: *Kali Sulph.*
Neuralgia occurring at night: *Calc. Phos.*
  periodic: *Mag. Phos.*, *Nat. Mur.*
  relieved by gentle motion: *Kali. Phos.*
    pleasant excitement: *Kali. Phos.*
  worse in cold weather: *Nat. Mur.*
    the morning: *Nat. Mur.*
Trembling hands: *Mag. Phos.*

SKIN

Blisters, with clear watery contents: *Nat. Mur.*
Burns: *Kali. Mur.*
  when suppurating: *Calc. Sulph.*
Burning, as from nettles: *Calc. Phos.*
Chapped hands from cold: *Calc. Fluor.*
Colourless, watery vesicles: *Nat. Mur.*
Cracks in palms of hands: *Calc. Fluor.*
Dry skin: *Calc. Fluor.*, *Kali. Sulph.*
Eruptions with watery contents: *Nat. Mur.*
  thick, white contents: *Kali. Mur.*
Excessive dryness of skin: *Nat. Mur.*
Exudations, when white and fibrinous: *Kali Mur.*
  albuminous: *Calc. Phos.*
  causing soreness and chafing: *Nat. Mur.*, *Kali. Phos.*
  clear, transparent, thin like water: *Nat. Mur.*
  greenish, thin: *Kali. Sulph.*
  mattery, or streaked with blood: *Calc. Sulph.*
  very offensive smelling: *Kali. Phos.*
  when pus is thick, yellow: *Silica.*
  yellowish and slimy,or watery: *Kali. Sulph.*

yellow, with small, tough lumps: *Calc. Fluor.*
   like gold: *Nat. Phos.*
Face full of pimples: *Calc. Phos., Calc. Sulph.*
Greasy scales on skin: *Kali. Phos.*
Hard, callous skin: *Calc. Fluor.*
Heals slowly: *Silica.*
Herpetic eruptions: *Nat. Mur.*
Inflammation of skin, for fever and heat: *Ferr. Phos.*
Itching, as from nettles: *Calc. Phos.*
   of skin, with crawling: *Kali. Phos., Calc. Phos.*
Mattery scabs on heads of pimples: *Calc. Sulph.*
Moist scabs on skin: *Nat. Sulph.*
Nettle-rash, after becoming overheated: *Nat. Mur.*
Perspiration, lack of: *Kali. Sulph.*
Pimples, with itching: *Calc. Phos.*
   under beard: *Calc. Sulph.*
Pustules on face: *Silica, Kali. Mur.*
Scaling eruptions on skin: *Calc. Phos., Kali. Sulph.*
Shingles: *Kali. Mur., Nat. Mur.*
   nervous symptoms: *Kali. Phos.*
   for the pain: *Ferr. Phos.* (powder applied locally), *Mag. Phos.*
Skin, festers easily: *Calc. Sulph.*
   hard and horny: *Calc. Fluor.*
   heals slowly and suppurates easily after injuries: *Silica.*
   dry, hot and burning, lack of perspiration: *Kali Sulph.*
   itching and burning, as from nettles: *Calc. Phos.*
   scales freely on a sticky base: *Kali. Sulph.*
   withered and wrinkled: *Kali. Phos.*
Stings of insects: *Nat. Mur.* (applied locally).
To aid desquamation in eruptive diseases: *Kali. Sulph.*
To assist in the formation of new skin: *Kali. Sulph.*
Ulcers around nails: *Silica.*
Yellow scabs: *Calc. Sulph.*
Warts: *Kali. Mur.*
   in palms of hand: *Nat. Mur.*
Wounds, do not heal readily: *Calc. Sulph.*
   neglected, discharge pus: *Calc. Sulph.*

FEVERS

Bilious fevers: *Nat. Sulph.*
Excessive exhausting perspiration, while eating: *Kali. Phos.*
Feeling of chilliness, especially in the back; watery saliva; heavy
    headache: *Nat. Mur.*
Fevers, vomit of sour fluids during: *Nat. Phos.*
  with chills and cramps: *Mag. Phos., Ferr. Phos.*
First stage of fevers: *Ferr. Phos.*
Increased thirst: *Nat. Mur.*
Inflammations, first stage: *Ferr. Phos.*
  second stage: *Kali. Mur.*
In eruptive fevers to aid desquamation: *Kali. Sulph.*
Perspiration, excessive: *Calc. Phos., Kali. Phos.*
  sour-smelling: *Nat. Phos., Silica.*
Profuse night sweats: *Nat. Mur., Silica, Calc. Phos.*
Shivering at beginning of fever: *Calc. Phos., Ferr. Phos.*
To assist in promoting perspiration: *Kali. Sulph.*

SLEEP

Constant desire to sleep in morning: *Nat. Mur.*
Drowsiness, with bilious symptoms: *Nat. Sulph.*
Great drowsiness in the elderly: *Silica.*
Hard to wake in morning: *Calc. Phos.*
Jerking of limbs during sleep: *Silica, Nat. Sulph.*
Nightmare, with bilious symptoms: *Nat. Sulph.*
Sleep does not refresh: *Nat. Mur.*
Sleeplessness from nervous causes: *Kali. Phos.*
Tired in morning: *Nat. Mur., Calc. Phos.*

AGGRAVATIONS AND AMELIORATIONS

Symptoms, aggravated:
  at night: *Silica., Calc. Phos.*
  by arising from sitting position: *Kali. Phos.*
  by change of weather: *Calc. Phos.*
    cold: *Nat. Mur., Calc. Phos., Mag. Phos.*
    cold air: *Mag. Phos., Silica.*

damp weather: *Calc. Phos., Nat. Sulph.*
draughts: *Mag. Phos.*
eating fish: *Nat. Sulph.*
fatty food: *Kali. Mur., Nat. Phos.*
getting wet: *Calc. Phos., Nat. Sulph.*
motion: *Ferr. Phos.*
noise: *Kali Phos., Silica.*
rainy weather: *Nat. Sulph.*
salty atmosphere: *Nat. Mur.*
touch: *Mag. Phos.*
in heated atmosphere: *Kali. Sulph.*
morning: *Nat. Sulph: Nat. Mur.*
evening: *Kali. Sulph.*
open air: *Silica.*
Symptoms ameliorated by:
bending double: *Mag. Phos.*
cold: *Ferr. Phos.*
cool air: *Kali. Sulph.*
eating: *Kali. Phos.*
excitement: *Kali. Phos.*
gentle motion: *Kali. Phos.*
heat: *Mag. Phos., Calc. Fluor.*
lying down: *Calc. Phos.*
pleasant excitement: *Kali. Phos.*

APPENDIX
Minerals and Trace Elements

Dr Schuessler was a pioneer in the realization of the importance of supplying the body with the right minerals in the right form to maintain good health and to correct ill-health.

Now nearly everybody recognizes the importance to health, growth and life of Calcium and Iron. It has also been discovered that some elements are dangerous in excess, especially Sodium in the form of common salt. We have begun to understand the importance of the so-called trace elements and it is generally realized that for complete health the body requires a supply of practically every inorganic element, mostly in very small quantities.

During the 50's and 60's the public became gradually aware of the importance of many vitamins to health, and it seems a safe prediction that throughout the 80's and 90's medical science will progress greatly in its knowledge of the function and value of trace elements, and this knowledge will be made known to the general public.

Meanwhile, there is enough information to give in this chapter a broad outline of the importance of the various minerals and trace elements drawing particular attention to those where deficiencies may arise. With this knowledge readers can consider for themselves whether they should take action to guard themselves against deficiencies by modifying their diet or by taking supplements, or both.

Calcium and Magnesium

The first two major minerals are Calcium and Magnesium. These are mentioned together because they work together in various ways, especially in maintaining the health of our bones and our muscles. They are very important indeed in maintaining the muscles of the heart in good condition.

Those of us who live in hard-water districts and drink tap-water probably get a good supply of both of these elements from that source. Dairy products such as milk, cheese and yogurt are a very valuable source of Calcium. Butter and cream do not provide very much as most of the Calcium is left behind in the skimmed milk. Skimmed milk powder, which can be used in cooking, in making yogurt, re-constituted as liquid milk etc., is a very valuable source of Calcium free of butter fat.

Vegetables are a good source of Magnesium especially if eaten raw. As a result vegetarians are unlikely to be short of Magnesium, but conversely vegans may be short of Calcium.

Fortunately, a very logical natural source of both Calcium and Magnesium is available in the form of Dolomite tablets. Dolomite is a mineral whose origin, like chalk, was in the laying down over millions of years of bones, shells, etc., of primitive creatures, and it has the important advantage that Calcium and Magnesium are present in it in the ratio of 1.65:1 which is exactly the same ratio as these elements are required in the body.

Iron

The next most important mineral to consider is Iron which, as everybody knows, is a vital constituent of blood, without which the blood cannot perform its essential function of transporting oxygen around the body. Lack of Iron eventually leads to anaemia.

Those of us eating a normal mixed diet including meats, and especially liver, probably get enough Iron. Vegetarians are at risk, especially vegans, unless they watch their diets very carefully making sure that they eat plenty of soya beans, dried fruits etc. Growing children and women of childbearing age have a larger requirement for Iron than the rest of us and are hence in danger of becoming deficient even on a normal mixed diet.

Iron supplements have been available for many years but unfortunately most of the earlier ones on the market were in forms which were poorly absorbed and could easily give rise to gastric irritation. Now, however, much improved Iron supplement tablets are available which provide this element in a form which is much more readily absorbed by the body and is less likely to cause gastric upsets. The best of these supplements are probably those where the Iron is present as gluconate.

Potassium and Sodium

The next two elements to be considered are Potassium and Sodium. Not only are both these elements required for the healthy functioning of the body but it is vital that we have them in the correct balance as it has been demonstrated that some people will develop high blood-pressure and other heart diseases if they have an excess of Sodium over a period of years.

We get most of our Sodium as common salt added to our food at the table and during the cooking process. Unfortunately, manufacturers also add Sodium, usually as common salt, to many processed foods during the course of manufacture. This is obvious in the case of products such as ham, bacon, etc., but perhaps not quite so obvious in very many other foodstuffs such as sausages, canned soups, butter, margarine, bread, etc.

The result of this is that anyone eating a normal Western diet will almost certainly be getting an excess of Sodium, probably a very large excess, unless they are making very strenuous efforts indeed to cut down on their salt intake. There is a great deal of very clear evidence of a direct link between the excess of Sodium in our diet and heart disease. For instance, the Belgians are very fond of ham, bacon and sausages of all kinds, and consume them in large quantities which results in a very high sodium intake. Over a period of time, however, they have developed more healthy eating habits and reduced their consumption of these salt-rich items. Happily, along with this reduction in salt intake, has come a reduced incidence of heart disease in Belgium.

We require rather more Potassium than Sodium in our diet, 2.5g per day as opposed to 2g per day of Sodium, and vegetables and fruits grown on soils containing a normal amount of Potassium are a good source. Unfortunately, food processing and cooking removes Potassium from our food with the result that it is estimated that only just enough Potassium for our needs is available in the average daily diet.

This is bad news for two reasons. One, if the average amount available is only just sufficient inevitably some of us are not getting enough. Also as we have seen the balance between Sodium and Potassium is important and as most of us are getting too much Sodium in our daily diet and only just enough or too little Potassium a very great number of us have a potentially dangerous ratio of Sodium t Potassium in our diet.

The first symptoms of a Potassium deficiency are a lack of energy strength and drive generally. Unfortunately, an excess of Sodiur both absolutely and in relation to Potassium does not show itself a once but possibly after some years in the form of high blood-pressur and heart disease.

What can we do about this? Well, first of all, all of us should b doing all we can to reduce the amount of Sodium in our diet. It i so omnipresent in our food as common salt that it is very unlikel that we will succeed in overdoing this unless we are living permanentl or temporarily in a very hot climate or engaged in an occupation suc as a steel foundryman, or doing very strenuous sports, or in any othe situation when we may lose a great deal of salt in the form c perspiration. In these comparatively rare situations we may actuall have to supplement our salt intake. In any case, we have our inbuil physiological craving for salt which will help us to avoid the unlikel risk of our becoming deficient in Sodium.

Potassium is another matter. As we have already seen, unless w are eating plenty of raw fruits and vegetables the chances are tha we are barely getting enough Potassium or are actually deficient i this element. Two questions arise, first, is it dangerous to have a excess of Potassium, and second, how can we set about addin; Potassium to our diet? To answer the first, there is probably no dange in a moderate excess of Potassium in the diet, but if we decide t take a Potassium supplement it is important which one we choos — more on this later.

There is even some evidence which suggests that as most of us ar getting far too much Sodium and are thus to a certain extent at ris from the point of view of high blood-pressure and heart disease, a moderate excess of Potassium may well have the beneficial effect o countering this.

This can be inferred from the results of a recent study in whicl young healthy males on normal diets were given Potassiun supplements in quantities equivalent to their normal total daily requirement. In other words, if their diet was already providing then with the required amount of Potassium, their total intake followin; the addition of the Potassium supplement was double their norma requirement. In this admittedly short test no adverse effects were seen but significant reductions in blood-pressure were achieved.

How do we go about getting sufficient Potassium? Well, farmers put Potassium on their fields in the form of manufactured fertilizers, so most raw vegetables and fruits are a good source of Potassium. Bananas and oranges are a good source but if you looked to these fruits for your total requirement of Potassium you would have to eat ten bananas or ten oranges a day to make sure of your total requirements. This will probably be too much of these particular fruits for most people.

Potassium supplements are available on the market but should be treated with caution. One type of tablet is made so as to release the Potassium slowly into the digestive system but unfortunately this type of tablet produces gastric irritation which can be dangerous. The other type is an effervescent tablet which is dissolved in water which is then drunk. This type of supplement avoids the problem of gastric irritation and makes the Potassium immediately available to the body instead of slowly over a period of time as would be the case when digesting a Potassium-rich food. The effervescent type of supplement is probably safe for most people to take providing no more than one tablet per day is taken immediately before or after a meal. Anyone in doubt, and this includes anyone with blood-pressure, heart disease or kidney problems, should consult a doctor before taking a Potassium supplement.

Trace Elements

We have so far considered five important metallic elements which are required by the body in quite significant quantities. We now come on to the question of trace elements which are required by the body in minute amounts, but nevertheless essential for complete health. The list of these trace elements is surprisingly long and includes virtually all the inorganic elements.

There are some surprises in this list! Arsenic, long known as a deadly poison, is in fact essential to the body in very minute quantities. Fortunately, there is Arsenic in our food and water in very minute amounts and a person with an Arsenic deficiency would be by way of being a curiosity. Thus we do not have to face up to the rather frightening prospect of trying to add more Arsenic to our diet!

The list of the trace elements which we require is a long one and includes Cobalt, Fluorine, Iodine, Nickel, Tin, Vanadium and quite a host of others. All are vital, but fortunately most of them we can get in one way or another in sufficient quantities from what we eat and drink. Tea for instance is a good source of fluorine and liver, kidneys and fish are good sources of most trace elements.

There are, however, five vital elements where there is definite evidence of wide-spread deficiencies. These are as follows:

1. *Chromium.* This is essential for the maintenance of correct blood sugar, and a deficiency may be associated with certain types of heart disease.
2. *Copper.* This is an essential part of various enzyme systems and a deficiency may well contribute to anaemia but an excess can be dangerous.
3. *Selenium.* This is beginning to be regarded as playing a valuable role in protection against cancer, and has recently shown to be of value to sufferers from arthritis.
4. *Zinc.* Probably the most important of all. It plays an essential part in more than forty of the body's vital enzyme systems and is crucial for healthy growth. Symptoms of a deficiency include depression, loss of appetite, poor or reduced sex drive and loss of taste and/or smell.
5. *Manganese.* This element is necessary for many vital processes including liver metabolism, the control of nervous irritability and the utilization of Vitamin C.

We tend to become deficient in these four elements because our food is now grown on soils that by successive cropping have been depleted of these minerals and it is not a normal farming practice to put them back in the form of fertilizers. There are further losses in the cooking and processing of food, and vegetarians, particularly vegans, are especially at risk because the two richest sources of virtually all the trace elements are liver and fish.

Fortunately, supplements including Zinc and Manganese as gluconates and Selenium and Chromium as yeasts are available as a combined tablet with or without Iron. Also for those identified as deficient in copper a tablet containing Zinc and Copper gluconate in an optimum ratio is available.

I will sum up this chapter by trying to answer two questions. How do I go about making sure that I and my family do not suffer from mineral or trace element deficiency? And how do I know if I have succeeded?

To answer the first, there are a few simple rules which help greatly:

1. If you are fortunate enough to live in a hard-water area (I say fortunate because it has been demonstrated very clearly that mortality from heart disease is much lower in hard-water areas than soft), make sure that you and your family drink tap-water and use tap-water for cooking and making beverages such as tea or coffee. If you have a water softener it is fine to use softened water for bathing, washing clothes etc., but do not drink it. The valuable Calcium and Magnesium have been removed and sinister Sodium introduced in their place.

2. Unless you do live in a very hot climate, engage in very considerable physical exertion, or otherwise are one of the very few where Sodium depletion through excessive perspiration is a danger, do your very best to reduce the amount of salt you take at table, use in cooking or take in the form of processed foods.

3. Eat a mixed diet containing as little as possible animal fat but with an emphasis on natural unprocessed foods, uncooked fruits and vegetables and cereal products. Non-fat dairy products such as skimmed milk and cottage cheese and liver and fish are also very valuable sources of minerals and trace elements. If you are a vegetarian or vegan I respect your convictions but would point out to you that you do have to watch your diet very carefully or take supplements to avoid deficiencies of Iron, and Calcium and the trace elements.

4. Finally, comes the matter of supplements:

    Dolomite tablets. These are a very logical, natural and safe source of both Calcium and Magnesium — and you need have no hesitation in taking them in the recommended dosage if you think you may have a deficiency of either Calcium or Magnesium.

    Potassium. Unfortunately, many of us are deficient in Potassium and/or have an adverse Sodium/Potassium balance. If you suspect this is the case you can eat oranges and bananas or take a Potassium supplement. Provided the correct supplement is chosen, i.e., the effervescent tablet which is drunk in the dissolved state. The taking of a Potassium supplement when required by persons in normal health and strictly following the dosage directions should present no problems.

Iron.   Safe and effective Iron supplements are now available and anyone particularly at risk of an iron deficiency, especially women of childbearing age or strict vegetarians, should have no hesitation in taking an iron supplement if they feel they need it.

Trace elements.   As we have seen, we need a large number of trace elements in our diet but fortunately, one way or another, we get an adequate supply of most of these. It does seem, however, that many people may tend to be deficient of one or other of the elements Zinc, Manganese, Chromium, Copper and Selenium. Fortunately, these are now available as tablets in an easily assimilable form in one tablet, with or without Iron.

Finally, how do you know whether you and your family are getting all the minerals and trace elements that they should? If your normal diet is more or less as has been described above, and particularly if you are taking the supplements recommended where any doubt exists, all is probably well. Your best confirmation of this will come if everyone in your family if full of health and vitality and resistant to minor infections.

If, however, all is not well and you still have doubts there is now a valuable check in the form of hair analysis. It has long been known that the minerals circulating in our blood stream are laid down in our hair and finger nails. This fact has been used in forensic medicine to detect the presence of Arsenic in the hair. Over the past few years the technique of hair analysis has been greatly improved as a means of seeing whether we have mineral deficiency, especially of trace elements.

If you wish to take advantage of this service you may be interested to know that the first totally British facility has recently been established in London by New Era Laboratories Ltd. at 39 Wales

Farm Road, North Acton, London W3 6XH, utilizing the experience and guidance of Dr P. Barlow of Aston University, Birmingham. This is no more expensive than other systems on offer which have to go to America for analysis, is perhaps even more advanced than some American systems and is much quicker in getting the results back to you. *New Era* will analyze your hair sample for you using a very modern computerized system and will send you a report which will show you how the mineral and trace element content of your hair compares with normal, and also warn you if the levels of any toxic metals such as lead or mercury are too high.

If this indicates any marked problem you can take corrective action either by modifying your eating habits or by taking appropriate supplements. Unfortunately, this service is not available on the N.H.S. Details are, however, available in most Health Food Stores.

General Index